THE FIRST YEAR OF LIFE

THE FIRST YEAR OF LIFE

FOURTH EDITION

H B VALMAN MD, FRCP
Consultant paediatrician,
Northwick Park Hospital,
Harrow, Middlesex

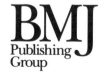

BMJ
Publishing
Group

First edition 1980
Second impression 1982
Second edition 1984
Second impression 1987
Third impression 1988
Third edition 1989
Fourth edition 1995

British Library Cataloguing in Publication Data

A catalogue record for this book is available from the British Library.

ISBN 0-7279 0897 9

Typeset in Great Britain by Apek Typesetters Ltd, Nailsea, Bristol
Printed and bound in Great Britain by Eyre & Spottiswoode, Margate

Contents

FOREWORD TO THE FIRST EDITION

The care of infants and their mothers has changed rapidly in the past 10 years and it is often difficult to identify those advances that will prove of lasting value to the clinician.

Dr Bernard Valman's articles on the first year of life, published recently in the *BMJ* and collected in book form, aim at providing the clinician in the community and in hospital with generally accepted views on the medical management of infants.

The main difference between paediatrics and general medicine is the range of normality, which changes with age. The greatest changes occur in the first year of life. Dr Valman's articles provide an account of normal development during this year, with particular emphasis on its assessment, so that deviations may be easily recognised. These articles have been collected together to provide a practical guide for general practitioners and the many other staff who care for the new born and young infants.

Stephen Lock
Editor, *BMJ* 1980

PREFACE TO THE FOURTH EDITION

The First Year of Life was the first series of ABC articles commissioned and published weekly by the *BMJ* and later collected and published as a book. The ABC series is continuing to tackle new subjects in all branches of medicine and surgery, and the original format has not changed. In 1979, when the first articles appeared, the *BMJ* was printed in black and white, but for this new edition of the book colour has been introduced, which enhances both the photographs and drawings. Each chapter has been thoroughly revised, especially the chapters on early prenatal diagnosis, resuscitation of the newborn, jaundice, diarrhoea and convulsions. There is a new chapter on failure to thrive. The chapters on surveillance and growth have been updated to include methods of collecting information for the parent-held record and the latest growth charts. The chapter on weaning includes recent recommendations of the Department of Health.

The book was written for family doctors, GP vocational trainees, medical students, midwives and nurses. It has become the standard textbook for several undergraduate and postgraduate courses. The emphasis has been on the practical aspects of management, based on clinical experience, but theory is introduced where it is essential for understanding the basis of management. No previous experience of paediatrics is assumed.

I wish to thank the staff of the *BMJ* and especially Deborah Reece and Barbara Horn, who have acted as midwives for the fourth edition of the book, and my wife who has constantly supported me and encouraged me to write.

For ease of reading and simplicity a single pronoun has been used for both feminine and masculine subjects; a specific gender is not implied.

EARLY PRENATAL DIAGNOSIS

Screening

- Ultrasound: 18–20 weeks
- Serum α fetoprotein: 16–18 weeks
- Mother over 37 years
  (a) Amniocentesis: 14–15 weeks
  or
  (b) Chorionic villus biopsy: 8–12 weeks

First antenatal visit

- Full blood count
- Group
- Rh antibody titre
- Rubella antibody titre
- Test for syphilis

Recent advances in ultrasound techniques and molecular biology have increased the range of antenatal diagnoses. Some methods are available only at specialised centres. This chapter will give a background to the successful techniques. An anomaly may be detected during routine examination of the fetus which is carried out by ultrasound in most pregnancies at 18–20 weeks of gestation. At present in some districts all mothers have a serum α fetoprotein (AFP) estimation as a screening test for neural tube or other defects and in all districts mothers of more than a certain age, usually 37 years, are offered amniocentesis or a chorionic villus biopsy to exclude Down's syndrome. The most effective methods of screening for Down's syndrome are being assessed and changes will be introduced shortly (see below).

After the birth of an abnormal baby or the detection of genetic disease in an older child, a paediatrician or geneticist may recommend a specific test at a particular week in the subsequent pregnancy. Some tests are at an early stage in development and the false positive and negative rates have not been assessed. Some genetic tests are not yet sufficiently precise to enable an accurate prognosis to be given to every family with that disease.

At the first antenatal visit it is still important to carry out a full blood count, blood grouping, rhesus antibody titre, rubella antibody titre, and a test for syphilis. Where indicated, haemoglobin electrophoresis may show that the mother has a haemoglobinopathy, and the father's red cell investigations may suggest that further studies of the fetus are needed.

Ultrasound studies

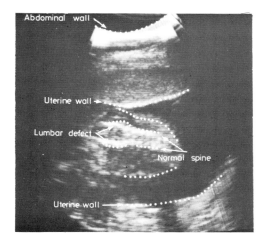

The first routine examination of the fetus by ultrasound is usually performed at the gestational age of 18–20 weeks. The gestational age is confirmed and anomalies of the central nervous system, kidneys, heart, intestinal tract, and skeleton are sought and may be detected. The consultant obstetrician, ideally with the paediatrician, should discuss the diagnosis and prognosis of an anomaly with both parents. Termination of the pregnancy may need to be considered, or serial ultrasound is performed during the pregnancy and in the neonatal period.

Ultrasound guidance has been used in taking samples of the chorion and amniotic fluid, and in selected centres it has been used to take blood samples from the umbilical cord (cordocentesis) and to give blood transfusion by that route. The blood samples can be used in gene probe techniques, enzyme estimation, and chromosome studies. In rhesus incompatibility a low haematocrit in the cord blood indicates the need for fetal transfusion. Cordocentesis has also been used in the assessment of renal function and oxygen transport in the fetus with intrauterine growth retardation.

Amniocentesis

Amniotic fluid is removed by passing a needle into the amniotic cavity through the mother's abdominal wall and uterus. Amniocentesis yields amniotic fluid with cells that have been shed from the skin of the fetus. Amniocentesis is performed when screening has shown a raised maternal plasma α fetoprotein concentration. A raised concentration of α fetoprotein is found in the amniotic fluid when the infant has

Early prenatal diagnosis

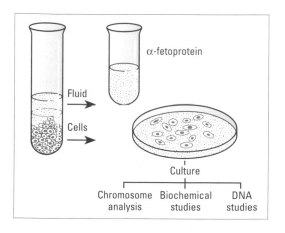

anencephaly or myelomeningocele. The levels of various enzymes can be measured in the fluid and are abnormal if the fetus is affected—for example, by cystic fibrosis. Examination of the cultured cells reveals the chromosome constitution of the fetus, including the sex; specific enzymes can be sought and deoxyribonucleic acid (DNA) probes used.

Many centres are carrying out amniocentesis at an earlier gestational age, such as 14–15 weeks, with good results. Some units have carried out amniocentesis earlier than this, but the earlier this is done, the fewer desquamated fetal skin cells are in the liquor and the higher is the failed culture rate. In one or two centres amniofiltration has been employed, where liquor is removed by amniocentesis at 10–12 weeks and filtered to remove desquamated fetal skin cells and then the liquor is returned to the amniotic cavity. It is too early to know whether this will become widely used in future.

Chorionic villus biopsy

Examples in which DNA gene probes are available

Autosomal dominant
- Huntington's chorea
- Myotonic dystrophy
- Adult polycystic kidneys
- Tuberous sclerosis
- Von Recklinghausen's disease

X linked
- Duchenne muscular dystrophy
- Haemophilia A and B
- Fragile X

Autosomal recessive
- α and β thalassaemia
- Sickle cell disease
- Cystic fibrosis
- Phenylketonuria
- α 1 anti-trypsin deficiency
- Congenital adrenal hyperplasia

Chorionic villus biopsy may be carried out by the transvaginal or, less commonly, by the transabdominal route under ultrasound guidance. The main indications have been maternal age, previous chromosomal anomaly, fetal sexing, enzyme assay, and gene probe assessment. Gene probes have been developed for several diseases including cystic fibrosis, Duchenne muscular dystrophy, and the haemoglobinopathies. DNA is extracted from the chorion sample and the probe is used to determine whether a specific part of a particular gene is present or absent.

Recent reports from the Canadian Multicentre Study and the UK Medical Research Council study confirmed the higher miscarriage rate with chorionic villus biopsy compared to amniocentesis. There was also a report of limb reduction deformities and facial abnormalities when chorionic villus biopsy was done early, transabdominally. These, together with a confirmed increase in the number of false positives and the introduction of early amniocentesis, have resulted in a swing away from chorionic villus biopsy to early amniocentesis. Chorionic villus biopsy is now reserved for women with high risk of congenital malformations.

Maternal serum used to screen for Down's syndrome

Criteria for amniocentesis	Detection of Down's syndrome (%)
>37 years	33
>37 years and all women with low α fetoprotein	45
>37 years and triple test positive	60–65

If all women over 37 had an amniocentesis, about one third of Down's syndrome babies would be detected. If all those women identified as being at risk by age together with women of all ages who have a low α fetoprotein had an amniocentesis, approximately 45% of Down's syndrome babies would be detected.

With the introduction of the triple test at 16–18 weeks gestation for *all* mothers, three biochemical parameters (serum α-fetoprotein, β-human chorionic gonadotropin (HCG), serum oestriol) are taken together with maternal age to improve the quality of risk assessment. If all those women identified as being at risk (screen positive = risk greater than 1:250) using the triple test had an amniocentesis, then it is thought that 60–65% of Down's syndrome babies would be detected. It is hoped that with the addition of ultrasound to detect soft signs such as an increase in nuchal thickness, dilated renal pelves or choroid plexus cysts, it may be possible to improve the risk assessment even more. In early pregnancy fetal cells can be detected in the maternal circulation in a ratio of about 1 000 000:1. It is hoped that in future, with improved techniques of DNA gene replication, it might be possible to karyotype a fetus from fetal cells in the maternal circulation.

Risks

The risk to a particular fetus depends on the gestational age of the fetus, the indication for the procedure, and the experience of the operator. The incidence of complications has fallen as skill in the newer techniques has increased. The abortion rates are difficult to assess, but the table opposite has been compiled from expert advice on the available evidence. The risk of abortion after amniocentesis at 15 weeks is about 1%, which is about twice the spontaneous incidence in normal pregnancies. Fetal or maternal bleeding has been considerably reduced by the use of ultrasound, but a slight risk of infection remains and the incidence of respiratory distress syndrome and orthopaedic problems, such as club foot, is probably slightly increased in fetuses who have undergone early amniocentesis. Chorionic villus biopsy has a higher risk of abortion of about 5% against a background of spontaneous abortion of 3%. Cordocentesis has a risk of about 2%. Chorionic villus biopsy carried out at about 10 weeks gestation provides a result early in pregnancy, when termination of the pregnancy is less traumatic and more acceptable for many mothers. Some tests are slightly more accurate when the sample is obtained by amniocentesis or cordocentesis. Some investigations can be performed only on specific samples.

Procedure	Gestational age performed (weeks)	Spontaneous abortion (%)	Risk of abortion after procedure (%)
Amniocentesis	14–15	0.5	1
Chorionic villus biopsy	9–12	2–3	3–5
Cordocentesis	18–20	<1%	1–2%

Screening for bacterial vaginosis

Preterm labour is the major cause of death and disability in babies. The aetiology of preterm labour is multifactorial but there is increasing evidence to implicate infection as a possible cause in up to 40% of cases. This information may not be of help once a woman is admitted in preterm labour, since by that time there may be irreversible changes in the cervix. Where the information may be of help is in the prediction and prevention of preterm labour. A few recent studies have reported that abnormal colonisation of the vagina in the form of bacterial vaginosis carries a risk of up to fivefold for the subsequent development of preterm labour and late miscarriage. Whether by reversing this condition it is possible to reduce the incidence of preterm labour and delivery is currently being tested.

RESUSCITATION OF THE NEWBORN

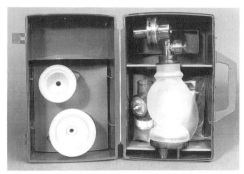

Resuscitation kit in case.

Wherever babies are delivered there should be a person with adequate skill and experience in resuscitation immediately available throughout the 24 hours. Most babies can be resuscitated with a closely fitting mask and an inflatable bag with a valve. The equipment is cheap, simple to use, and can be carried in a small case. Some infants cannot be resuscitated by this method but require intubation, which to be successful should be done by a doctor or midwife with continual experience of the procedure.

Babies who have developmental brain abnormalities before labour may develop fetal distress during the stress of labour and may have difficulty in establishing spontaneous respiration. For this reason, the contributions of brain development and perinatal management in the causation of later cerebral palsy is often difficult to resolve.

Assessment

	0	1	2
Appearance (colour)	Blue, pale	Body pink, extremities blue	Completely pink
Pulse (heart rate)	Absent	Below 100	Over 100
Grimace (response to stimulation)	No response	Grimace	Cry
Activity (muscle tone)	Limp	Some flexion in extremities	Active movements
Respiration (respiratory effort)	Absent	Slow irregular	Strong cry

The following high risk factors indicate that resuscitation may be needed:

- fetal distress
- caesarean section
- preterm infant
- breech delivery
- forceps delivery
- twins
- maternal anaesthetic
- maternal diabetes
- rhesus incompatibility

These factors predict about 70% of the babies needing resuscitation. The remainder arise unexpectedly. The APGAR scoring system is used to assess the infant's condition one minute and five minutes after birth. A numerical score is given for each of five features. The heart rate and respiratory effort determine the action to be taken.

Procedure

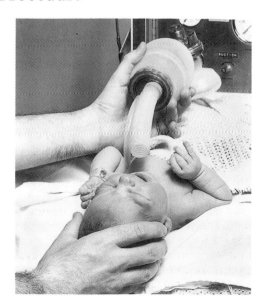

Suctioning the oropharynx

It is best not to use mucus extractors, as there is a risk of the operator swallowing or inhaling infectious material. Use a suction catheter (size FG 8) connected to the Resuscitaire or directly to a wall suction unit. The mouth can safely be suctioned but care must be taken in the oropharynx. This should be done under direct vision and is usually part of tracheal intubation. Do not blindly push the catheter as far as it will go since this can cause a vagally-mediated bradycardia and apnoea and is invariably associated with a fall in oxygen saturation.

Administering facial oxygen

Set the oxygen flow rate to 5 l/min and hold the funnel-shaped mask just in front of the baby's face. The oxygen may be connected either to the funnel-shaped mask or to the bag and mask apparatus, but in the case of the latter, it is prevented from flowing out of the mask by the valve unless the bag is compressed. However, it will come out of the corrugated tube that is attached to the other end of the bag, so turn it round and hold the end of this tube to the baby's face.

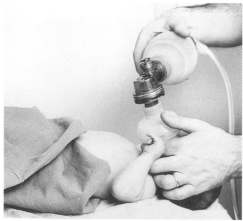

Operator holding mask with *right* hand to show how to extend infant's head.

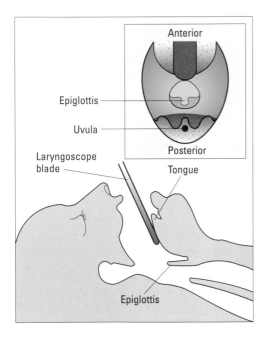

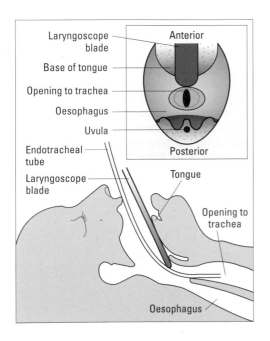

Using the bag and mask

If the infant does not breathe by 30 seconds after birth, the closely fitted mask is applied to the face with the head extended. The left hand is used to hold the mask to the baby's face while the right hand squeezes the bag. Place the little and ring fingers of your left hand under the baby's chin and with gentle traction slightly extend the neck. This prevents the head from moving around and straightens the upper airways, ensuring their patency. With the other fingers and thumb, apply the mask firmly to the baby's face to ensure a tight seal. A proper seal is confirmed when you squeeze the bag, as there is a characteristic rasping noise as the valve opens. If the seal is inadequate, the valve makes no noise and you will not feel any resistance when squeezing the bag. This can be practised with the mask against the palm of your hand. Use only the thumb and two fingers, rather than your whole hand, to squeeze the bag. Do not empty the bag but gently depress it to a few centimetres only. This will safeguard against a pneumothorax. The smaller the baby, the gentler you must be. The rate should be maintained at 40/min with an inflation time of approximately 1 second. Check you are producing an adequate chest expansion. Air is usually used but oxygen can be introduced into the bag through a side arm.

Intubation

If there are no spontaneous respiratory movements at the end of one minute after birth or if the heart rate is less than 100 beats/min at any time the infant should be placed supine on a flat surface. A special resuscitation trolley is ideal. The laryngoscope is held in the left hand and passed over the infant's tongue as far as the epiglottis. The tip of the blade is advanced over the epiglottis about another 0·5 cm and is then withdrawn slightly. This presses the epiglottis against the root of the tongue, revealing the glottis. In the newborn the glottis is a slit in the centre of a small pink mound and the slit may expand into a triangular opening during a gasp. Gentle backward pressure on the infant's larynx by an assistant may help to bring the glottis into view. Secretions in the pharynx should be aspirated with a large catheter—for example, FG 9. The endotracheal tube held in the right hand is then guided through the larynx about 1 to 2 cm into the trachea.

Intermittent positive pressure should be applied at a rate of 40 times per minute with an inflatable bag with a valve.

The positive pressure applied should not usually be higher than 30 cm H_2O; otherwise there is a danger of rupturing the lung and producing a pneumothorax or pneumomediastinum. These low pressures are enough to induce a gasp reflex, which is then followed by normal respiratory movements of the chest. Occasionally in an infant with a severe lung problem, such as severe meconium aspiration or diaphragmatic hernia, higher pressures are needed. A return to a normal heart rate is a good sign that resuscitation is satisfactory. If the endotracheal tube has to be left in place for a short period the tube should be fixed to the cheek by adhesive tape.

Aspiration of secretion in the endotracheal tube and in the trachea can be carried out with a fine catheter (suction catheter FG 6). The shoulder on the endotracheal tube is designed to prevent the tube going too far down through the vocal cords and therefore into the right main bronchus, but this may still occur. If breath sounds are heard equally on both sides of the chest the tube is probably in the trachea and not beyond the bifurcation.

Intermittent positive pressure should be stopped every three minutes for about 15 seconds to determine whether spontaneous respiratory movements will start.

During prolonged apnoea the blood pressure is maintained initially but later falls. If the heart rate is less than 100/min a short period of cardiac massage should be given at the same time as efforts to start respiratory movements. Cardiac massage is carried out by applying firm pressure with two fingers over the lower sternum.

Hypothermia is a special hazard for infants who have been resuscitated and exposed during these procedures. Rapid initial drying of the infant with a warm towel is the most important preventive factor, but resuscitation should also be carried out under a radiant heater of at least 400 watts. After resuscitation, infants should be wrapped up and handed to their mother for at least a minute or two even if they have to be placed in a transport incubator and taken to the special care unit. Most full-term infants who have required resuscitation do not need to be admitted to the special care unit.

Failure to improve

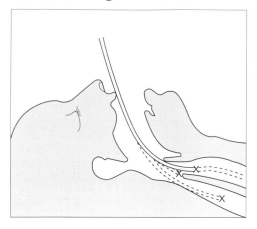

The best sign that resuscitation has been successful is an increase in heart rate. If this does not occur within about 15 seconds the following should be considered. (1) The gas cylinders may be empty or the pipe line disconnected. (2) The endotracheal tube may have been misplaced into the oesophagus or have slipped out of the trachea during extension of the neck. If there is any doubt the tube should be removed and a fresh tube inserted immediately. (3) The endotracheal tube may be in the right main bronchus. After these possibilities have been excluded other diagnosis to be considered are pneumothorax, pulmonary hypoplasia associated with Potter's syndrome (renal agenesis with a squashed facial appearance and large, low set floppy ears), and diaphragmatic hernia.

Drugs

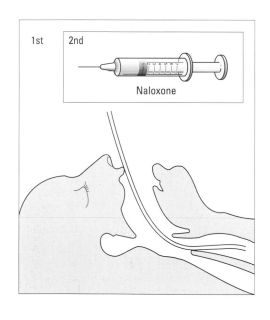

If the mother has recently received pethidine or morphine, a chemical antagonist can be given to the infant. If the infant needs both intubation and drugs, intubation should always be performed first. The only chemical antagonist available is naloxone, but its period of action is short. The manufacturer's current recommended dose is 10–20 micrograms per kilogram body weight, which can be given intramuscularly or intravenously and may be repeated at 2 to 3 minute intervals. Alternatively, a single dose of 60 micrograms/kg body weight may be given intramuscularly at birth.

An adequate supply of oxygen quickly reverses acidosis and it is rarely necessary to consider giving intravenous sodium bicarbonate or glucose solution.

If there are no spontaneous respiratory efforts by three minutes after starting resuscitation, blood is taken for urgent pH and bicarbonate estimations. Without waiting for the result, the probable acidosis is partially reversed by giving 4 ml/kg body weight of 2·1% sodium bicarbonate solution slowly at a rate that does not exceed 2 ml/min. The standard 8·4% sodium bicarbonate solution must be diluted 1 in 4 with sterile water for intravenous use. The solution should be given by a peripheral vein if possible, as the solution is hypertonic and may cause local vascular damage. If this is not possible, an umbilical vein catheter can be used in an emergency.

Ten per cent glucose solution can be given if a BM stix shows hypoglycaemia.

Adrenaline can be given if there is asystole or there is persistent severe bradycardia. If there is no response, sodium bicarbonate solution, followed by calcium gluconate can be given in the recommended doses. There is no evidence that adrenaline or calcium gluconate improve the prognosis. The infant is transferred to the neonatal intensive care unit.

There is no specific treatment for the hypoxic-ischaemic encephalopathy that may follow perinatal asphyxia. The infant may be apnoeic and need continuous positive pressure ventilation, have fits, episodes of bradycardia, lethargy, or be reluctant to suck. Mannitol, frusemide, steroids, and phenobarbitone in high doses have been used to prevent or treat possible cerebral oedema but there is no evidence that they are effective.

Recommended doses

Drug	Concentration	Route	Dose (ml/kg)	Dose for 3 kg baby (ml)
Adrenaline	1 in 10 000 (0.1 mg/ml)	IT*, IV, IC	0·1	0·3
Calcium gluconate	10%	IV	0·2	0·6
Sodium bicarbonate	8.4% (1 mmol/ml)	IV	1	3 (dilute 1 in 4 with water)
Glucose	10%	IV	1–2	3–6
Albumin	5%	IV	10–20	30–60
Atropine	600 micrograms/ml	IV, IT*	0·03	0·09
Naloxone HCl	20 micrograms/ml	IM, IV	0·5	1·5

* Double the dose and add 2 ml of 0·9% sodium chloride solution for intratracheal route

These infants will also need long-term follow-up to assess neurological development. The survival rate of full-term newborn infants who have taken 20 minutes to breathe spontaneously is about 50% and about 75% of the survivors are neurologically intact.

When to stop

Poor outcome can be predicted when spontaneous respirations are not established by 30 minutes. If, in addition, there is no cardiac output, then survival cannot be expected. It is at this stage that attempts at resuscitation should cease.

When not to start

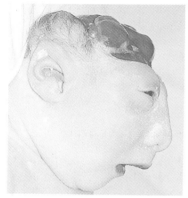

Anencephaly.

This can be an extremely difficult decision and should not be made by the most junior paediatrician, so begin resuscitation and call for help. If the heart rate has been recorded at any time during the second stage of labour, resuscitation should be attempted even if there is no heartbeat at birth. With fetal monitoring it is uncommon for babies to die during labour and stillbirths are usually expected. Babies who have been dead for longer than 12 hours have an obvious "macerated" appearance with gross peeling of the skin.

A baby born at less than 22 weeks gestation cannot survive and often a paediatrician will not be called if the obstetrician is sure of the dates. Certain conditions are non-viable, such as anencephaly or gross hydrocephalus, but fortunately these are usually detected prior to birth and a decision is reached with the parents before delivery.

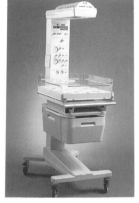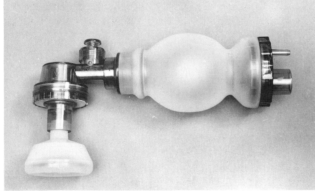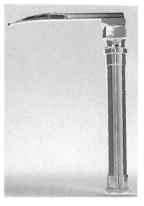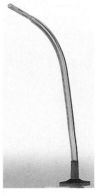

From left to right: resuscitation trolley (reproduced by kind permission of Vickers Medical); bag with face mask; small laryngoscope with straight 10 cm blade; neonatal endotracheal tube.

Vitamin K

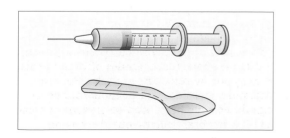

Vitamin K is given to all babies as prophylaxis against haemorrhagic disease of the newborn. The dose is 1 mg for full term babies and 0·5 mg for preterm infants. A single intramuscular dose protects against the early form of haemorrhagic disease, which occurs between the second and fourth day, and the late form, which occurs after three or four weeks. Recent controversy on the safety of the intramuscular route has resulted in some units prescribing several oral doses (although the preparation is not yet licensed in the UK), but I recommend that the intramuscular route should be used at present as blood levels are more predictable.

Discussion with parents

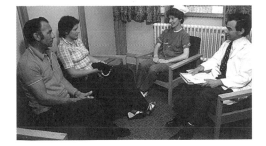

An infant who is breathing normally should be given to the mother after a rapid examination. She should be told that the infant seems to be normal and that it is common for infants to need help with breathing at birth. It is important to emphasise that the infant's progress will be no different from that of other infants who have not needed resuscitation. Most infants who have required intubation should go with their mothers to the postnatal wards and receive routine observation. Only if there has been a prolonged period before the establishment of spontaneous respiration should the infant be taken to the special care unit.

If resuscitation has not been successful, the person responsible for resuscitation, together with a member of the obstetric staff, should see both parents immediately. The parents should be asked whether they would like to see the dead infant, who should be suitably wrapped up before being brought in to them. A nurse is usually with the parents to answer questions about the baby's appearance. The mother may be anxious to hold the baby, and if so it may be kinder to leave her alone to grieve over her dead baby for a few minutes. Discussion with the parents will help to decide who is the best person to help them with their grieving and with the reactions of the other children in the family. The family doctor should be told by telephone as soon as possible.

INFANTS OF LOW BIRTH WEIGHT

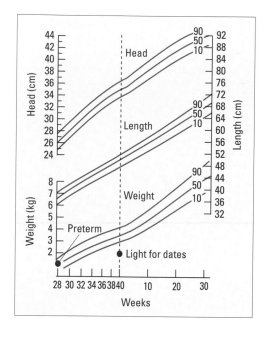

Low birth weight infants weigh 2500 g or less at birth. Infants may be small at birth owing to a short gestation period (born too early) or because of a retarded growth rate. When the period of gestation is less than 37 completed weeks the infant is called preterm. A baby with retarded growth rate is "light for dates" and may be either malnourished or rarely hypoplastic (for example, an infant with a chromosome abnormality). Some babies who are preterm are also light for dates.

The length of gestation, as calculated from the first day of the mother's last menstrual period, can be confirmed by the routine ultrasound examination carried out at 18 weeks. Detecting retardation in growth of the fetus is difficult, but palpation of the fetus can be supplemented by serial measurements of the fetal skull, abdominal girth, femur length and crown rump length.

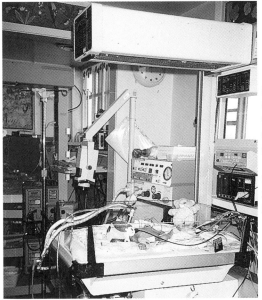

The gestational age of the infant can be assessed by a detailed neurological examination of the infant, as the development of the central nervous system is related to the gestational age. Scoring systems using both the neurological development and specific external features can be used to estimate the gestational age within an accuracy of about a week.

Most neonatal units consider that infants with a birth weight below the tenth centile for the gestational age are light for dates, although a more accurate definition is below the third centile with an adjustment for maternal size.

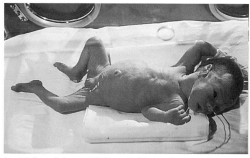

Ultrasound studies have shown that when intrauterine malnutrition starts early in pregnancy the head circumference and weight are in proportion with each other, but when malnutrition starts late in pregnancy the head is disproportionately large, owing to relatively normal growth of the brain.

The preterm infant is especially prone to developing hypothermia, the respiratory distress syndrome, infection, and intracranial haemorrhage. The light-for-dates infant is particularly prone to hypothermia, hypoglycaemia, and hypocalcaemia.

Light for dates: 1800 g at 40 weeks

Temperature

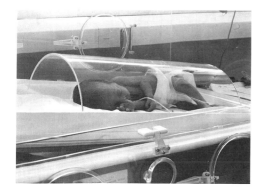

Small infants become hypothermic quickly. Heat loss may be considerable because they have a large surface area in relation to body weight and they are also deficient in subcutaneous fat, which provides insulation. They also lack "brown fat", which is usually present in a full term baby and can be metabolised rapidly to produce heat.

Hypothermia is associated with a raised metabolic rate and increased energy consumption. To prevent hypothermia small infants should be kept in a high constant environmental temperature. Excessive heat loss by radiation can be minimised by an additional tunnel of perspex, a heat shield, placed immediately over an infant in an incubator. The dangers of hypothermia can be reduced by carrying out resuscitation under a heat lamp or radiation heat canopy, bearing in mind the danger of burns if the lamp is too close. When an infant is transferred from one hospital to another for special care, there is a danger of hypothermia. A swaddler made of aluminium foil has been designed to prevent this and is commercially available, but wrapping the baby with Gamgee wool is also satisfactory.

The portable incubator must be kept warm continuously and ready for immediate use.

Infection

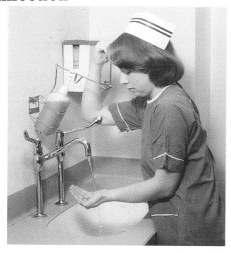

Nurses who are scrupulous about washing their hands are probably the most important factor in preventing cross infection. In many units medical and nursing staff no longer wear masks and gowns, though a separate plastic apron or waterproof gown should be used for nursing each infant, mainly to prevent soiling the nurses' clothes.

Scrupulous washing of the hands should be carried out before and after touching each infant. Washing with soap and water is adequate, although many units use a disinfectant soap solution. Scrubbing with a brush is unnecessary. Although this principle is simple, it may be difficult to ensure that it is carried out. Proper use of elbow taps is often difficult because of their poor design. Using disposable plastic gloves when changing infants' napkins may reduce cross infection.

Ideally, any infant who develops an infection should be barrier nursed in a separate cubicle.

Feeding

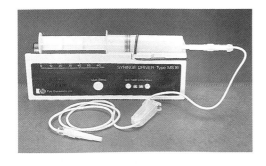

Preterm infants have poor sucking and cough reflexes, and methods of feeding must prevent aspiration into the lungs. Infants who are not able to suck are given frequent tube feeds of small volumes or continuous intragastric feeds to avoid sudden falls in arterial oxygen concentrations and apnoeic attacks, which are associated with abdominal distention. In many units transpyloric feeding using a weighted tube that passes into the jejunum has been used successfully, but it is technically more difficult. Intravenous feeding with glucose amino acid solutions and lipids is used for infants who do not tolerate tube feeding, but a scrupulous aseptic technique in managing the solutions is necessary to avoid septicaemia.

Early feeding, within two hours of birth, prevents hypoglycaemia and reduces the maximum plasma bilirubin concentrations. Asymptomatic hypoglycaemia can be detected early by performing regular Boehringer Mannheim (BM) stix tests on all babies with low birth weights every three hours. If the infant is feeding well and the BM stix tests consistently indicate blood glucose concentration above 2 mmol/l, the tests are stopped after 24 hours. From the second week onwards vitamin supplements are added so that infants receive an additional dose of 400 units of vitamin D and 50 mg of vitamin C daily. Vitamin preparations usually contain small amounts of vitamin B complex and vitamin A. Vitamin supplements should be given until the age of 2 years and additional iron supplements until the age of 6 months.

BREATHING DIFFICULTIES IN THE NEWBORN

Breathing difficulties in the newborn are called respiratory distress. One or more of the following features are present:

(a) respiratory rate over 60 per minute;
(b) an expiratory grunt;
(c) subcostal or intercostal recession or sternal retraction;
(d) cyanosis.

Respiratory distress syndrome

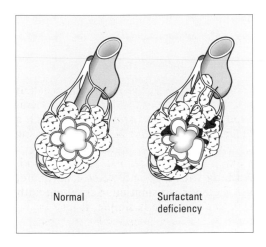

Normal   Surfactant
              deficiency

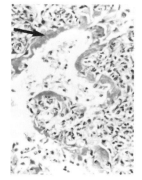

Arrow indicates hyaline membrane.

The respiratory distress syndrome is the commonest cause of respiratory problems in the newborn and a common cause of death in preterm infants. Cerebral ischaemia and haemorrhage, or lung damage may occur in the acute phase and cause death or long term morbidity. Hypoxia before, during, or after birth is a predisposing factor.

The cause is a deficiency of pulmonary surfactant, a substance normally present on the alveolar walls. Surfactant lowers the surface tension in the alveoli so that during the first few breaths the same pressure is required to inflate them all. This produces uniform inflation of all alveoli. Surfactant also prevents the alveolar walls from collapsing during expiration. Without surfactant the surface tension is great in the smaller alveoli, causing them to collapse, while large alveoli continue to expand easily. Thus there is uneven expansion, with increasingly widespread alveolar collapse. Surfactant production in the fetal lung increases with gestational age and reaches adequate levels for normal lung function by about the thirty-sixth week. At 27–31 weeks 35–50% of all infants are affected by the respiratory distress syndrome.

Microscopy of postmortem specimens often shows the presence of amorphous material lining the terminal bronchioles and alveoli, which is called hyaline membrane. There are also multiple areas of alveolar collapse.

When animal surfactant extract or artificial surfactant is placed in the trachea at birth or during the first day of life, the severity and mortality of the respiratory distress syndrome is reduced. Supplementary surfactant appears to be most effective in babies of more than 26 weeks of gestation. Supplementary surfactant is given at birth either to all babies within a specific range of gestation or to preterm infants who have developed specific features of surfactant deficiency that suggest that the course of the disease will be of moderate or greater severity (rescue treatment).

Clinical features and general management

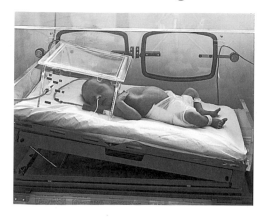

An expiratory grunt, a respiratory rate over 60 per minute, and recession of the chest wall begin within four hours of birth. Central cyanosis may appear later. Usually auscultation of the lungs reveals only reduced breath sounds, but crepitations may be present. The present approach to intensive care is to monitor the blood arterial oxygen, carbon dioxide, and pH levels from birth and to start treatment early. This may prevent the appearance of the features described above, especially where artificial ventilation is used electively from birth in infants weighing less than 1 kg.

In most infants the chest radiograph shows normal lung fields in the early stages of the disease, but later a fine reticular pattern or generalised loss of translucency (the ground glass appearance) may be present. The contrast between the air in the bronchi and the opaque

Breathing difficulties in the newborn

lung fields produces an air bronchogram. The greatest value of the chest radiograph is in excluding other conditions (see below).

The object of management is to support infants until further surfactant is produced. Infants should be handled as little as possible, as movement during frequent recording of rectal temperature or changing the sheet may make their condition deteriorate abruptly. Infants should be given oxygen, their arterial blood oxygen and carbon dioxide concentrations should be monitored, and body temperature, fluid and electrolyte balance maintained.

Management

- Temperature
- Arterial oxygen
- Carbon dioxide
- pH
- Blood pressure
- Plasma Na, K, creatinine

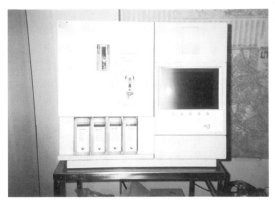

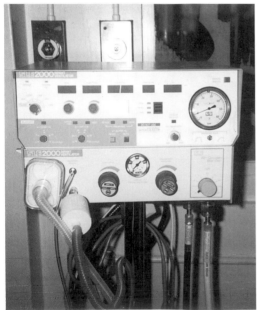

Blood oxygen analyser.

Oxygen treatment and measurement

During oxygen treatment the arterial oxygen tension should not fall below 6·7 kPa (50 mm Hg) or rise above 12 kPa (90 mm Hg). Below 6·7 kPa the risk of cerebral palsy and mental retardation increases, and above 12 kPa there is a possibility of retrolental fibroplasia and subsequent blindness. Some infants may need high concentrations of inhaled oxygen to prevent hypoxia. This can be given safely only if there are facilities for making frequent estimations of the blood oxygen concentrations.

The ideal arterial carbon dioxide level is 5–7 kPa (37·5–52 mm Hg). Lower carbon dioxide levels may cause cerebral artery constriction and reduce cerebral blood flow. Higher carbon dioxide levels may lead to cerebral artery dilatation followed by systemic hypotension or intraventricular haemorrhage.

There are several methods of measuring oxygen concentrations in the blood. Firstly, samples can be taken from an umbilical artery catheter at regular intervals or they can be obtained by repeated puncture of one of the radial arteries.

Secondly, an oxygen sensitive electrode implanted into the tip of an umbilical artery catheter measures oxygen levels continuously, but the electrode must be calibrated at regular intervals with samples of blood aspirated through the lumen of the same catheter.

Thirdly, a heated transcutaneous oxygen and carbon dioxide electrode increases the blood flow to the skin, where the gas tensions are measured. The electrode must be moved every four hours to avoid burns. The method is not invasive and the electrode is calibrated with a gas mixture. The levels shown by the transcutaneous electrode must be compared with levels estimated in arterial blood at regular intervals. The blood samples are also used to measure pH, bicarbonate and base deficit. `

Artificial ventilation

Results of artificial ventilation have improved considerably during the past few years and deaths are now usually due to complications rather than respiratory failure. Respiratory tract infection and displacement of the endotracheal tube are constant hazards and this form of treatment can only be undertaken where there are adequate nursing and medical staff, and enough patients for an effective service to be provided.

Positive pressure ventilation is needed if one of the following is present:

(*a*) failure to establish effective spontaneous respiration at birth;
(*b*) recurrent apnoeic attacks;
(*c*) Arterial oxygen tension (Pa_{O_2}) less than 7 kPa in 60% oxygen;
(*d*) Arterial carbon dioxide tension (Pa_{CO_2}) more than 7 kPa;
(*e*) rapid deterioration in blood gas values associated with clinical deterioration.

Ventilator.

Other aspects of treatment

Incubators are used to improve observation. There are two types—the conventional incubator and an open type. A perspex head box can be used to maintain an oxygen concentration above that in the air.

Adequate fluids and electrolytes must be given. The methods will vary with the severity of the respiratory problem. Milk can be given by continuous gastric or intrajejunal infusion. Alternatively, small volumes of milk can be given intermittently at frequent intervals. Some infants need intravenous fluids.

The group B *Streptococcus* may produce a clinical picture similar to that of respiratory distress syndrome, and infants with the respiratory distress syndrome need antibiotics. Intravenous antibiotics must be given until blood culture results are known, as the syndrome cannot be differentiated from group B streptococcal pneumonia in the early stages.

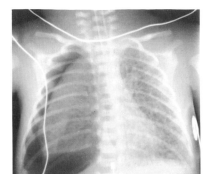

Pneumothorax.

Complications

A pneumothorax should be suspected in any infant who deteriorates rapidly for no obvious reason. The diagnosis may be confirmed quickly by transilluminating each side of the chest with a powerful fibreoptic light source. A chest x ray can be used to confirm the condition, but if symptoms are severe the pneumothorax can be drained before the radiograph has been obtained. A disposable cannula is inserted into the pleural space and connected to an underwater seal. Pneumothorax may also follow intermittent positive pressure ventilation during resuscitation of the newborn or it may occur as a result of the initial vigorous spontaneous respiratory efforts of a normal infant.

Cerebral lesions

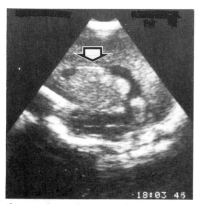

Arrow shows intraventricular haemorrhage.

Periventricular and intraventricular haemorrhage are the most common forms of intracranial haemorrhage in the newborn infant. The high prevalence of periventricular lesion is related to advances in neonatal intensive care, which have led to increased survival of the preterm infant. About 20% of the infants with birth weights less than 1500 g have shown evidence of this type of haemorrhage when ultrasound scans have been performed routinely within the first few days of life. These haemorrhages originate in the subependymal germinal matrix and may spread to involve the ventricular system or may extend into the cerebral parenchyma adjacent to the lateral ventricle. Most of the infants with periventricular haemorrhage have no specific symptoms but some infants have recurrent apnoeic attacks, impaired spontaneous limb movements, and hypotonia or sudden severe clinical deterioration. Small localised periventricular haemorrhages are associated with a good prognosis but early mortality is high and long term handicap is common in infants with extensive haemorrhages or periventricular leucomalacia. This condition is considered to be related to hypoxia and ischaemia of the brain and is shown by small cysts in the periventricular region in ultrasound scans of the brain taken after the third week of life. These lesions are associated with later major handicaps such as cerebral palsy, blindness, or deafness.

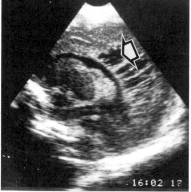

Arrow indicates periventricular leucomalacia.

Bronchopulmonary dysplasia

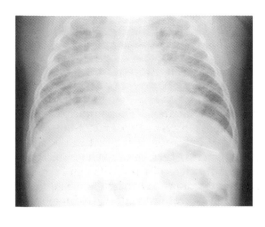

This is a chronic respiratory disease occurring in preterm babies who have needed prolonged artificial ventilation. Intermittent positive pressure ventilation is probably more important than oxygen treatment in the aetiology. The infant requires increased inflation pressures or ambient oxygen concentrations as coarse streaking and areas of hyperinflation appear on the chest radiograph after the first two or three weeks of life. After weaning from the ventilator, supplementary oxygen is often required for several months, and those with severe disease die usually about the third month of life. The survivors have a high prevalance of recurrent episodes of wheezing but usually have no further clinical respiratory symptoms after about 18 months of age. Dexamethasone started between the second and fourth week may reduce the respiratory support needed to prevent hypoxia. A transcutaneous oxygen saturation monitor is used to assess the effects of treatment.

Other causes of respiratory problems

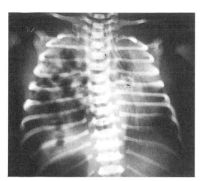

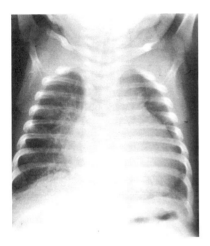

Diaphragmatic hernia.

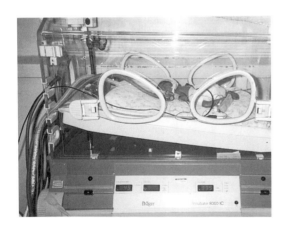

Large heart.

The main causes are pulmonary, cardiac and central nervous system disorders.

Transient tachypnoea of the newborn is found in full-term infants and usually resolves within 48 hours. The chest radiograph often shows a streaky appearance of the lung fields but may be normal. This syndrome may be due to failure of normal reabsorption of the lung fluid at birth or it may be a mild form of respiratory distress syndrome.

Diaphragmatic hernia may present with difficulty in resuscitating the baby or with a raised respiratory rate and an apex beat on the right side. The hernia is most commonly left sided and the heart is often displaced to the right. The diagnosis is confirmed by a chest radiograph that shows loops of small gut or solid organs in the thorax. It may take 12 hours from birth for air to reach the colon and produce the characteristic *x*-ray appearances.

The first symptoms of *congenital heart disease* are often noticed by the nurse or mother when the infant has dyspnoea during feeding or is reluctant to feed. There may be no murmurs with some lesions. The respiratory rate is raised and there may be recession of the chest wall. Excessive weight gain and enlargement of the liver are early confirmatory signs. The edge of the liver is normally about 2 cm below the costal margin in the right midclavicular line in the full term newborn.

Pneumonia may occur if there has been rupture of the membranes for longer than 24 hours: the infant may inhale infected liquor before birth and so develop pneumonia. If the mother has had ruptured membranes for over 24 hours before delivery antibiotics should be considered for the mother to prevent or treat pneumonia in the fetus.

Group B streptococcal infection may present with a raised respiratory rate, and a chest radiograph may show extensive areas of consolidation in both lungs or may appear normal.

Meconium aspiration usually occurs in an infant who has become hypoxic before delivery. The infant may start respiratory movements before the mouth and pharynx have been cleared. Aspiration of meconium may cause bronchial obstruction, secondary collapse, and subsequent infection of the distal segments of the lungs. In some units the high mortality has been reduced by bronchial lavage at birth, but this needs considerable skill. Oxygen and antibiotics are often needed and mechanical ventilation may be required for a few days.

Preterm infants have a poor cough reflex, and material such as regurgitated milk in the pharynx is easily aspirated into the lungs and may cause pneumonia. Signs may be minimal and are often limited to a small increase in respiratory rate, but a chest radiograph may show extensive changes.

Severe anaemia may cause a raised respiratory rate with a metabolic acidosis.

Choanal atresia or stenosis—a congenital posterior nasal obstruction makes it difficult for newborn infants to breathe, as they depend on a clear nasal airway. An oropharyngeal airway produces immediate improvement, and an ENT surgeon should be consulted. The diagnosis can be confirmed quickly by noting the absence of movement of a wisp of cotton wool placed just below the nares.

Apnoea

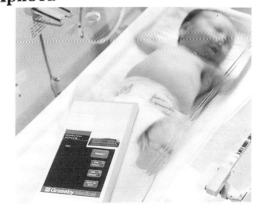

Apnoeic attacks are defined as episodes of cessation of respiratory movements for more than 10 seconds. They may be due to cerebral hypoxia during the perinatal period, hypoxaemia due to the respiratory distress syndrome, hypoglycaemia, or meningitis. An ultrasound scan of the brain may help in determining the presence and site of any intracranial haemorrhage.

Morphine or pethidine given to the mother before delivery may cause apnoea in the newborn (see page 6).

Recurrent apnoeic episodes are common in preterm infants of less than 32 weeks gestation. The babies are otherwise well and the episodes start when the infants are a few days old. The apnoea may be accompanied by bradycardia and a fall in transcutaneous oxygen saturation levels. Recent research suggests that some episodes are of central and others of laryngeal origin. The diagnosis of apnoea of prematurity can be made only after excluding other causes, which are:

(a) pulmonary disease,
(b) airway obstruction, for example due to aspiration of feeds;
(c) hypoglycaemia;
(d) hypocalcaemia;
(e) intracranial haemorrhage;
(f) convulsions, which may be misdiagnosed as apnoea;
(g) cardiac disease.

Several attacks may occur daily for the first month of life. These may be difficult to manage and may be followed by cerebral palsy at a later date if the episodes are prolonged. The various forms of treatment include stimulation of a limb during attacks or prophylaxis with aminophylline or continuous positive airways pressure.

Causes of apnoea

- Prematurity
- Hypoxia
- Intracranial haemorrhage
- Hypoglycaemia
- Meningitis
- Drugs

BIRTH TRAUMA

Cephalhaematoma

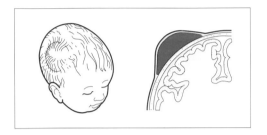

Cephalhaematoma is a subperiosteal haemorrhage that is limited by surrounding sutures. In most cases there is probably a hairline fracture of the underlying cranial bone, which may be difficult to demonstrate but is unimportant since it affects only the outer table. There is usually no brain damage. A surprisingly large amount of blood may be present and blood transfusion is occasionally required. The lesion may not be noticed until the third day.

During resolution a calcified rim may appear, which wrongly suggests a depressed fracture, or there may be a hard swelling that takes several months to disappear.

Cephalhaematoma must be distinguished from caput succedaneum, which is a soft-tissue swelling due to oedema of the part of the head presenting at the cervix and which is not limited by the sutures.

Chignon

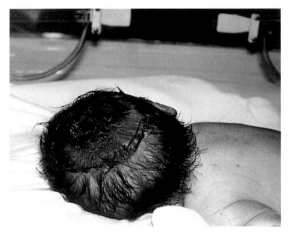

Vacuum extraction is often associated with a "chignon," which is subcutaneous oedema where the cap has been applied. In some cases a large haematoma may form and occasionally the skin becomes necrotic. Nevertheless, the skin grows rapidly from the borders to cover the area within a few weeks.

Fractures

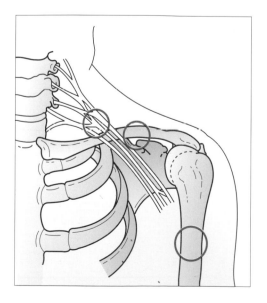

Fractures of the clavicle or humerus and stretching of the brachial plexus present as lack of spontaneous movement and an absent Moro reflex in the arm on that side. The clavicle and humerus should be radiographed. Fracture of the clavicle needs no treatment, but if the humerus is fractured the arm should be splinted to the infant's body with a crêpe bandage. Injuries to the brachial plexus sometimes have a poor prognosis and the infant should be seen by an orthopaedic surgeon for advice on preventing contractures. Diaphragmatic paralysis often accompanies stretching of the brachial plexus and may cause a raised respiratory rate. Another condition that may be mistaken for injury of the brachial plexus is temporary paralysis of the dorsiflexors of the wrist caused by pressure on the radial nerve in the radial groove of the humerus. A fracture of the humerus may injure the radial nerve at this site.

Intracranial injuries

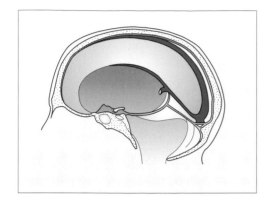

When the fetal head is large in relation to the pelvic outlet or delivery is precipitate or by the breech, there is a risk of extracerebral haemorrhage due to laceration of the tentorium cerebelli or falx cerebri affecting a venous sinus.

Infants may be unduly lethargic or especially irritable shortly after birth, and there are usually no helpful confirmatory signs then. Later there may be pallor, a high pitched cry, poor muscle tone or increased tone, convulsions, reluctance to suck, vomiting, or apnoeic attacks, and fast or periodic breathing. Rarely the tension of the anterior fontanelle is raised, the heart rate is slow, or the pupils fail to react to light. A BM stix test should be performed to exclude hypoglycaemia, a plasma calcium concentration estimated, and a lumbar puncture considered to exclude meningitis.

Infants should be nursed in an incubator for easy observation but if they weigh over 3000 g, the thermostat should be turned to the minimum level. This type of haemorrhage is now rare. The prognosis is poor.

Other conditions

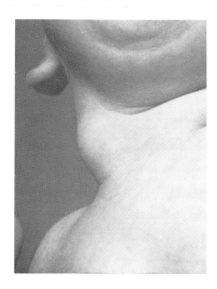

A sternomastoid "tumour" is not noticeable at birth but usually presents after the first week. A firm mass, 1–2 cm in diameter, is usually found in the middle or lower third of the sternomastoid muscle but it may be anywhere along its length. It will disappear within a year and usually the infant will then be perfectly normal. The mother is taught by a physiotherapist to move the infant's head passively through the whole range of normal movements daily until the lesion resolves. Without treatment about 10% of the infants develop torticollis in the second year of life and a further 10% when they are over 5 years old.

Subconjunctival haemorrhages, like petechiae on the head and neck, are common and unimportant. But if there are petechiae on the trunk further investigations are indicated.

Subcutaneous fat necrosis produces a firm subcutaneous area at the site of pressure, especially of the obstetric forceps. It may be red and tender. No treatment is needed. If the site is unusual and the swelling not noticed until a few days after birth, the area of necrosis may be confused with a pyogenic abscess.

Pressure on the facial nerve before birth or from obstetric forceps may cause a transient palsy which lasts up to two weeks. Care of the exposed cornea is essential.

SOME CONGENITAL ABNORMALITIES

Myelomeningocele

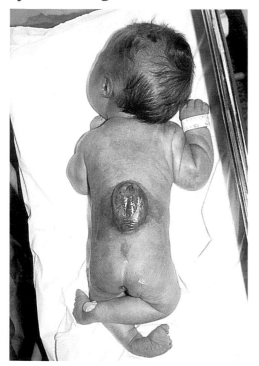

A myelomeningocele is a flat or raised neural plaque partly devoid of skin in the midline over the spine due to abnormal development of the spinal cord and associated deficiency of the dorsal laminae and spines of the vertebrae. It is usually found in the lumbar region. The absence of the various coverings that normally protect the cord allows meningitis to occur easily. If there are no active movements in the legs and the anus is patulous, the infant will probably be incontinent of urine and faeces for life and never be able to walk unaided. Thoracic lesions and kyphosis are signs of poor prognosis.

Infants with a good prognosis need urgent treatment, so all affected infants should either be seen by a consultant paediatrician without delay or sent to a special centre, where selection for surgery can be made. About 30% of the infants have surgery as a result of this policy. During the first operation the lesion on the back is covered by skin.

Most of these infants develop progressive hydrocephalus later and those considered suitable for surgery require insertion of a catheter with a valve from a cerebral ventricle to the peritoneal cavity to reduce the cerebrospinal fluid pressure.

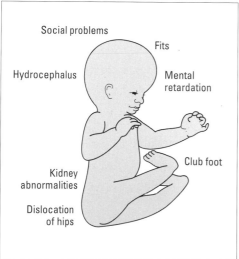

Hydrocephalus can be detected by ultrasound examination of the brain. Serial measurements show whether ventricular size is increasing rapidly. In addition, progressive hydrocephalus is confirmed by measuring the circumference of the head at its largest circumference (occipitofrontal) every three days with a disposable paper tape measure, plotting these values on a growth chart, and showing that the head is growing faster than normal.

Raised concentrations of α fetoprotein are found in the amniotic fluid when the fetus has an open myelomeningocele or anencephaly. In anencephaly there is absence of the cranial vault and most in the brain. In some units *maternal plasma* α fetoprotein levels are measured in all mothers at the 16–18th week of gestation. An ultrasound examination is performed and the *amniotic fluid* concentration is estimated in the mothers with a raised plasma value who wish to have these investigations and are prepared to have a termination of an affected pregnancy.

Microcephaly

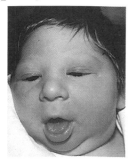

The signs of microcephaly are a small head and forehead that is particularly small in relation to the face. The diagnosis is confirmed by showing a small head circumference in relation to the baby's weight and gestational age. It is invariably associated with mental impairment. Other congenital abnormalities may be present. Evidence of an intrauterine infection such as toxoplasmosis should be sought to enable the parents to receive accurate genetic counselling.

Cleft lip and palate

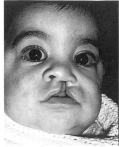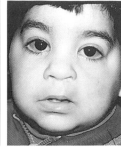

Mothers are often severely disturbed by the appearance of these infants and may be reassured by seeing photographs of similar patients before and after their repair operations. Cleft lip and cleft palate are often associated. A cleft lip, caused by failure of the maxillary process growing towards the midline to fuse with the premaxilla, may be unilateral or bilateral. Minor degrees of cleft palate may be easily missed if the posterior part of the palate is not seen and palpated. Most of these infants feed normally from the breast or bottle. If there are feeding difficulties, a special teat, a large normal teat, a special spade-like spoon, or an ordinary spoon may be tried. The lip is usually repaired at three months and the palate at one year. The value of an obturator before operative closure of the palate is controversial. If an obturator is needed, it should be made and fitted within 24 hours of birth. Despite excellent operative results these children are prone to recurrent otitis media and problems with speech development.

Umbilical hernia

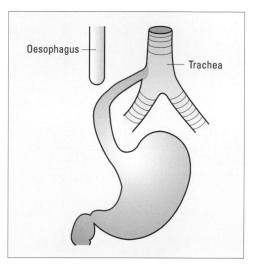

An umbilical hernia, usually containing omentum and gut is most common in African infants or West Indians of African descent. No treatment is needed, as the hernia usually disappears spontaneously by the age of 3 years, although in West Indian infants it may take a further three years.

In contrast to an umbilical hernia, the sac of an omphalocoele is covered by peritoneum but incompletely by skin. An omphalocoele is a hernia into the base of the umbilical cord and contains gut and sometimes solid organs like the liver. Immediate transfer to a surgical unit is needed.

Oesophageal atresia

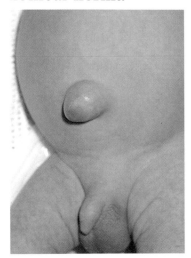

Oesophageal atresia will be suspected in any newborn baby who has a continual accumulation of frothy secretions in the mouth with drooling, sometimes with cyanotic attacks.

The diagnosis of oesophagal atresia is confirmed by attempting to pass a tube down the oesophagus. The tube should have a relatively wide lumen (FG 10), must be stiff enough to prevent coiling in the upper oesophageal pouch, and should have a radio-opaque line so that the position can be checked by a chest radiograph. The tube should be aspirated every few minutes to keep the upper pouch clear until the infant reaches a specialised surgical unit.

Multiple abnormalities

Infants with multiple abnormalities should be examined and investigated by a paediatrician without delay to ensure correct management *of the infant* and to provide the information needed for genetic counselling. Some of the infants may have a recognisable syndrome and the investigations may show a chromosomal defect or evidence of intrauterine infection.

Some congenital abnormalities

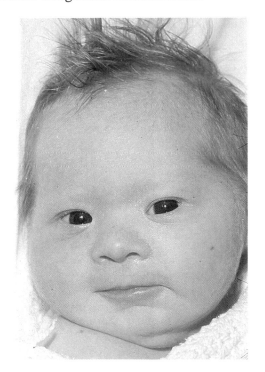

The most common problem is the infant with possible Down's syndrome (mongolism). Although a scoring system for a large number of clinical features has been used it the past, any infant with suspected Down's syndrome should have a blood chromosome analysis performed. The most useful features suggesting the diagnosis are the facial appearance with palpebral fissures that slant upwards and outwards, prominent epicanthic folds, baggy cheeks, and white spots on the iris. A flat occiput, poor limb tone, and single palmar crease are suggestive but not specific signs. About 2% of normal infants have a single palmar crease in one hand, and prominent epicanthic folds are even more common. If the infant has congenital heart disease, it may be detected by performing an ultrasound study, as a definite murmur may not be present until several weeks after birth. All infants with Down's syndrome have developmental delay, but it may be possible to reduce maternal depression and increase the infant's drive and ability to learn by introducing the parents to an occupational therapist in the neonatal period.

ROUTINE EXAMINATION OF THE NEWBORN

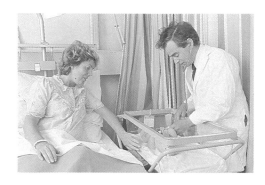

Immediately after birth all infants should be examined for the presence of gross congenital abnormalities or evidence of birth trauma. Later, preferably on the morning after delivery, every infant should be examined again in detail. The obstetric notes should be checked to determine whether the infant has been at special risk—for example, from maternal rubella or a difficult delivery. A systematic approach should be used so that abnormalities are not missed. The infant must be completely undressed and in a good light. The mother should be present during the examination so that the results of the examination can be discussed with her and so that she can voice her anxieties.

Skin

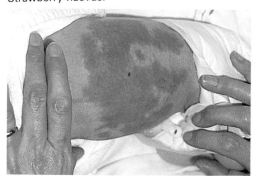

Strawberry naevus.

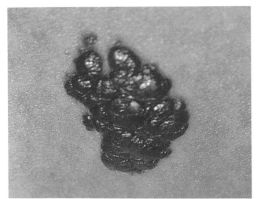

Port wine stain.

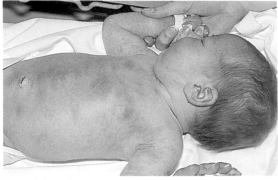

Neonatal erythema.

Diffuse capillary naevi on the face, eyelids, or occiput are common and resolve within a few months.

The "strawberry mark" starts as a tiny red spot and grows rapidly for several weeks until it has a raised red appearance with small white areas, suggesting the seeds of a strawberry. Such marks are common in preterm babies. They may occur anywhere on the body but cause no symptoms, except on the eyelids, where they may prevent easy opening of the eyes and need treatment. Strawberry naevi grow, often rapidly, for three to nine months, but at least 90% resolve spontaneously, either completely or partially. Resolution usually begins at 6 to 12 months and is complete in half the children by the age of 5 and in 70% by the age of 7 years. In 80% of cases these naevi resolve completely without trace.

The port wine stain is not raised and may be extensive. It does not resolve, but the skin texture remains normal. When the naevus occurs in the distribution of the trigeminal nerve, there may be an associated intracranial vascular anomaly.

Neonatal erythema (erythema "toxicum") consists of blotchy ill defined areas of bright erythema surrounding white or yellow wheals which may resemble septic spots. It usually appears on the second day of life and in most infants clears within 48 hours. The lesions contain many eosinophils and have no pathological importance. Neonatal erythema is more common in full-term infants. By ringing individual lesions with a skin pencil they can be shown to disappear in a few hours, to be replaced by others elsewhere. This contrasts with septic lesions, which appear later and do not resolve so quickly.

Mongolian blue spots are patchy accumulations of pigment, especially over the buttocks and lower back in infants of races with pigmented skins. They are common in babies of African or Mongolian descent, but also occur in Italian and Greek babies. They may be mistaken for bruises and a wrong diagnosis of non-accidental injury made. They become less obvious as the skin darkens.

A midline pit over the spine is most commonly found over the coccyx, where it does not usually communicate with the spinal canal. A midline pit anywhere else along the spine may be connected with an underlying sinus, which may communicate with the spinal canal and requires excision to prevent the entry of bacteria and meningitis.

Head and neck

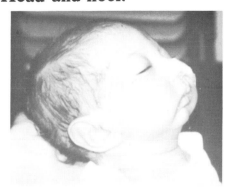

An infant with the Pierre Robin syndrome has a small lower jaw, glossoptosis, and cleft palate. The infant must be nursed prone to prevent his tongue falling backwards and occluding the airway. A small jaw may occur alone or with other abnormalities. As the child grows the small size of the lower jaw becomes less obvious.

Nodules of epithelial cells resembling pearls (Epstein's pearls) just lateral to the midline on the hard palate are a normal finding. A cluster of these pearls is present at the junction of the hard and soft palates.

Heart murmurs

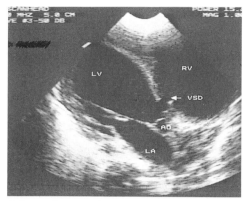

Echocardiogram showing ventricular septal defect (VSD).

In the first two days of life one of the most common problems is an infant who is feeding normally but is found to have a short systolic murmur during a routine examination. The murmur is usually due to a patent ductus arteriosus and has usually disappeared by the time the infant is examined again at 7 days. An electrocardiogram (ECG) or chest radiograph is unnecessary.

If a long murmur is first heard around the eighth day of life, a chest radiograph, ECG, and echocardiogram should be performed and the infant seen by a paediatrician. Most of these murmurs are due to a ventricular septal defect or mild pulmonary stenosis with no symptoms. Most of the ventricular septal defects (VSD) close spontaneously before the infant reaches the age of 5 years.

The normal respiratory rate at rest is less than 60/min, and there should be no recession of the chest wall or below the mandible. If there is any murmur and the infant is feeding poorly or has a respiratory rate faster than 60/min at rest, a chest radiograph and ECG should be performed and the baby seen by a paediatrician urgently. These symptoms and signs indicate congestive heart failure usually due to multiple heart defects.

Cyanosis of the hands and feet has no importance if the tongue is of normal colour and the infant is feeding normally.

Abdomen

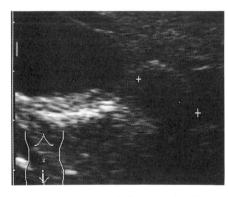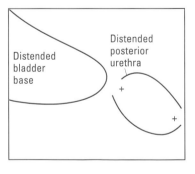

Ultrasound scan and diagram showing distended bladder and distended posterior urethra due to urethral valves.

The liver edge is normally 1–2 cm below the costal margin in the midclavicular line. In a thin, relaxed infant the kidneys may be palpable bimanually.

The inguinal areas are inspected for the presence of a hernia. Absence of the femoral pulses suggests that coarctation of the aorta is present. The blood pressure is measured in all four limbs and the advice of a cardiologist is obtained urgently.

Failure to pass urine in the first 36 hours or a poor urinary stream suggests posterior urethral valves in a boy. An enlarged bladder may be palpable. Diagnosis is confirmed by an ultrasound examination, which may show hydronephrosis and cysto-urethrogram.

Patency of the anus is confirmed by inspection.

Genitalia

The foreskin is attached to the penis at birth and no attempt should be made to retract it.

A hooded prepuce suggests hypospadias with the urethral orifice at the base of the glans penis. If the urethral meatus is adequate, no immediate treatment is needed, but the infant must not be circumcised and should be referred to the plastic surgeon's next clinic.

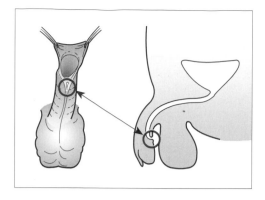

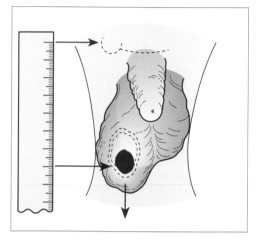

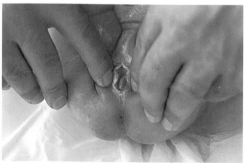

Vaginal mucosal prolapse.

If the urethral orifice is nearer the perineum, the adrenogenital syndrome should be considered. In the adrenogenital syndrome cortisol secretion fails and the adrenals produce excessive androgen. Girls become virilised, with enlargement of the clitoris and fusion of the labia and may be mistaken for boys (see page 53). In boys the genitalia are normal.

Intersex is a less common cause of ambiguity of the external genitalia, and a paediatrician should be consulted without delay. An accurate diagnosis is an emotional and social emergency. The parents should be advised that the baby should not be named until the results of chromosome studies are available.

Small hydrocoeles usually disappear spontaneously during the first month but an associated inguinal hernia should be sought.

Poor development of the scrotum suggests that an undescended testis is present. Undescended testis is especially common in preterm infants, in whom the testes usually descend during the first three months after birth. An undescended testis is present in 30% of preterm and 3% of term infants at birth. An infant with an undescended testis should be seen again at the age of 3 months. At that time 5% of preterm infants and 1% of term babies will still have an undescended testis and they should be referred for surgery, which is performed at about the age of 2 years. If the baby develops an associated hernia, the operation will be needed as an emergency.

As the cremasteric reflex is usually absent at birth, the testis cannot be retractile. If there is any doubt about whether a testis is descended the examiner should (a) palpate the pubic tubercle with one hand, (b) hold the testis between the thumb and forefinger of the other hand and gently draw it down to its fullest extent, then (c) measure the distance from the pubic tubercle to the centre of the firm globular testis.

At term the testis, if fully descended, lies 4–7 cm from the tubercle. If the distance is under 4 cm the testis has not completely descended. In preterm babies, who are more likely to have undescended testes and whose testes are smaller, 2·5 cm has been arbitrarily chosen to divide descent from non-descent.

In girls a small amount of vaginal bleeding is common, usually five to seven days after birth, and follows excretion of maternal or placental oestrogens, which are transmitted to the fetus before birth. White vaginal discharge or prolapse of the vaginal mucosa is normal.

In either sex physiological enlargement of the breast may occur towards the end of the first week. This enlargement, which may be unilateral, resolves within a few weeks, but if there is local redness, a breast abscess should be suspected.

Club foot and extra digits

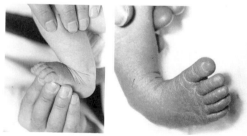

Postural.   Structural.

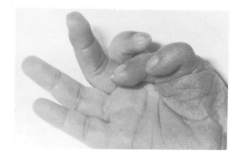

Muscular imbalance due to the posture of the infant's feet in utero is the commonest cause of club foot. In postural club foot it should be possible to dorsiflex the foot fully and to obtain passive inversion to 90°. The mother should be taught to manipulate the foot through the whole range of movements after each feed for several days after birth, although the shape usually reverts to normal within a few weeks even without treatment. In contrast, in structural club foot the range of passive movements is restricted, and orthopaedic advice on strapping, manipulation, or serial plasters is needed within 24 hours of birth.

To detect extra digits, the digits should be counted with the infant's palms open, or an extra thumb may be missed. Polydactyly requires the advice of a plastic surgeon to determine which digit should be removed at the age of 3 or 4 years for the best functional results. Extra fingers and toes are often familial and vary from an apparently normal digit to a skin tag. The latter can be tied off with a sterile silk thread and will separate by aseptic necrosis.

Central nervous system and eyes

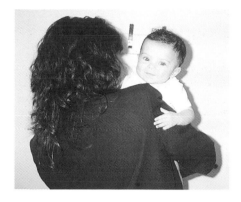

To assess the central nervous system the alertness of the infant and the symmetry of spontaneous movements should be noted. The tension of the anterior fontanelle and the width of the fontanelle should be palpated while the infant is at rest, and the head circumference should be measured. A more detailed neurological examination is not required unless there is a special indication.

Babies will open their eyes when being fed or when held upright over their mother's shoulder. Babies will follow the movements of an examiner's face provided that the distance is 50 cm or more. The pupils of every baby should be examined with an ophthalmoscope at a distance of 50 cm. A bright red glow is seen, which is a reflection of light from the back of the retina. Absence of this "red reflux" is found in congenital cataract, which produces a dull grey appearance.

Phenylketonuria and hypothyroidism

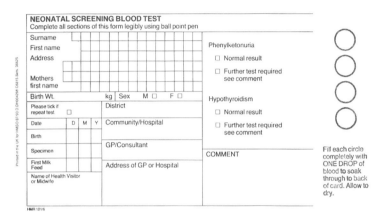

The Guthrie test detects high blood concentrations of phenylalanine, which indicate that the infant probably has phenylketonuria. Drops of blood are taken by heel prick after six days' breast or bottle feeding (usually the seventh day of life) and placed on the special absorbent card provided. The blood is usually taken by the health visitor if the infant is at home on the seventh day. If the test is positive, the infant should be admitted to hospital to confirm the diagnosis, as he or she may need a special low phenylalanine diet to prevent brain damage. In some areas a capillary tube of blood is collected (for the Scriver test) instead of the dried-blood spot.

Some laboratories use the plasma thyroid stimulating hormone and others the plasma thyroxine value as the screening test for hypothyroidism. The screening blood card is used for both the Guthrie test and the test for hypothyroidism.

Talking to parents

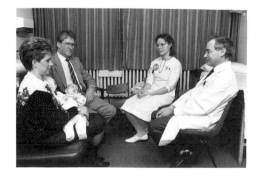

Whenever possible both parents should be seen together. If an abnormality is found during the routine examination some indication must be given to the mother so that arrangements can be made to see both parents. Particularly if the problem is likely to be long term, the doctor who will continue the long-term care should speak to the parents initially. Ideally, a nurse should be present as well since the parents will probably ask all the questions again as soon as the doctor has left.

The diagnosis should be explained in terms that the parents can understand, and the positive aspects should be emphasised. For example, if the probable diagnosis is ventricular septal defect, it is not necessary to explain that there is a remote possibility of multiple cardiac defects. After a difficult forceps delivery it is better to say that most babies develop normally rather than say they may be slightly backward. An unnecessarily pessimistic prognosis based on out-of-date information may alter a mother's attitude towards her baby and impair her attachment to him or her.

In discussing management the help and support that will be given by social workers or physiotherapists should be emphasised and the parents advised to tell their relations and friends the diagnosis rather than hide it.

A doctor with only limited experience of a particular problem should tell the parents that he or she needs to seek further advice rather than guess at the answer. Parents often cling to the first opinion and may find it difficult to accept a more experienced view later. A statement of the facts—for example, that there is an abnormality of the spine—may be given with the assurance that a more experienced doctor will discuss them later.

Birth details

Please use ball point pen and press firmly

Date of birth _____ / _____ / _____

Time of birth _____

Weeks of pregnancy _____

Method of Delivery _____

Place of birth _____

Problems during pregnancy or birth:

(1) _____

(2) _____

(3) _____

(4) _____

Meconium passed within 24 hrs	Yes/No
In special care baby unit	Yes/No
Any neonatal contraindication to immunisation	Yes/No
Risk factors for congenital dislocation of hip	Yes/No
Risk factors for hearing loss	Yes/No/Not Known
Feeding at discharge	breast/bottle/both

Blood tests done

Phenylketonuria	Yes/No	Norm/Abn
Thyroid test	Yes/No	Norm/Abn
Haemoglobinopathies	Yes/No	Norm/Abn

For office use:
White copy: keep in Record   Yellow copy: to Child Health Office
Pink copy: to GP/HV   Green copy: for hospital record (with sticky strip on reverse)

Infant Hospital No. _____

Birth Wt. _____ kg   Head circ. _____ cm

Apgar at 1 & 5 mins _____

(Tick box if examination done and write in 'comments' if problem)

Comments

Skull sutures	☐	_____
Skin	☐	_____
Eyes – Red reflex	☐	_____
Palate	☐	_____
Heart	☐	_____
Abdomen	☐	_____
Genitalia	☐	_____
Hips	☐	_____
Limbs/Spine	☐	_____

Significant abnormality or condition _____

_____

_____

Follow-up hospital appointment   Yes/No

Reason/details _____

_____

_____

Birth details

Immunisations

ALL CHILDREN SHOULD RECEIVE IMMUNISATIONS except a very few children who:
1. are suffering from a feverish illness – when the immunisation should be postponed until full recovery.
2. have had a severe reaction to a previous immunisation (see 'Help and advice' section for mild upsets page 24).
2. have an illness or are taking medicines that interfere with their ability to fight infections.

CHILDREN TAKING ANTIBIOTICS CAN BE IMMUNISED.
Before each immunisation the doctor or nurse will make sure that it is all right to give your child the vaccine.

Further comments on consultation sheets: YES/NO

Please use ball point pen and press firmly

Age due	Site of injection	Vaccine	Date given	Batch Number	Signature in full	Treatment Centre Code
Dose 1 2 months	RL/LL ..... RL/LL	*D.T.P. or *D.T. Polio Hib				
Dose 2 3 months	RL/LL ..... RL/LL	*D.T.P. or *D.T. Polio Hib				
Dose 3 4 months	RL/LL ..... RL/LL	*D.T.P. or *D.T. Polio Hib				
12 months		Measles, Mumps Rubella (MMR)				

*Delete one

For office use:
White copy: keep in Record
Yellow copy: to Child Health Office

Immunisations

DISLOCATED AND DISLOCATABLE HIP
IN THE NEWBORN

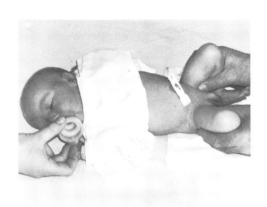

Congenital dislocated hip and dislocatable hip are probably the most important asymptomatic congenital abnormalities to detect, as early treatment is simple and usually effective. In the first 12 hours of life 10 in 1000 infants in Britain have a hip abnormality. When the examination is carried out 24–36 hours after birth the incidence falls to about seven per 1000 births. Formerly, when they were all left untreated in the newborn, the incidence of established dislocated hip was 1 in 800 children. There may be a family history of the condition; the anomaly is more common in girls and after the extended breech position in utero. There is a higher incidence in some countries, such as Italy and the former Yugoslavia.

The best time to examine the infant's hips is between the ages of 12 and 36 hours, as the tendency to provoke regurgitation is less by that time. The examiner's hands should be warm and the infant should be placed on her back with the sheet spread completely flat. She should be fully relaxed, and this may be encouraged by putting an empty sterile feeding teat in her mouth if necessary. The gentle abduction test, followed by Barlow's test, should be carried out in all cases. Unnecessary trauma to the delicate hip joint and its capsule must be avoided.

Gentle abduction test

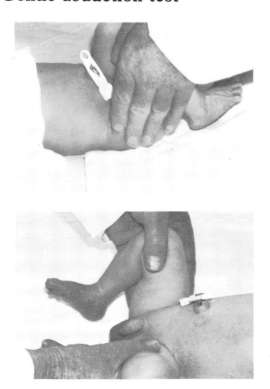

The gentle abduction test will detect hips that are in the dislocated position at rest. Each hip should be examined separately, while the opposite thigh is gently fixed by the examiner's other hand. Both the knee and the hip should be flexed to a right angle and the knee held so that the examiner's thumb is parallel to the medial aspect of the lower thigh, while the middle two fingers lie along the whole length of the lateral aspect of the femur. The tips of the examiner's fingers thus lie over the greater trochanter.

The thigh should be held *lightly* and neither pushed down towards the cot surface nor pulled up towards the examiner's face. It should then be allowed to abduct very gently and slowly by the weight of the infant's leg until abduction is complete. The thigh should never be forcibly abducted and it is unnecessary to obtain abduction beyond 10° above the flat. While abducting the thigh, the examiner may feel or see the head of the femur slip, jerk, or jolt forward into the acetabulum. A temporary interruption in the flow of abduction at a point about midway through abduction precedes the sensation of this abnormal movement of the head of the femur.

If the joint capsule is very lax, the reduction jolt may be missed unless great care is taken.

Barlow's test

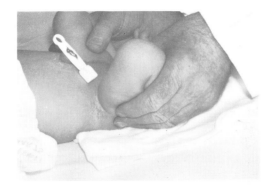

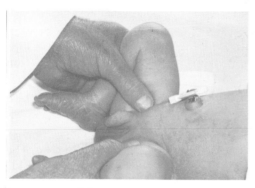

The object of Barlow's test is to identify dislocatable hips in which the head of the femur can be gently jolted posteriorly over the posterior lip of the acetabular labrum to lie temporarily out of the acetabulum and those dislocated hips in which the head of the femur can be jolted forwards to lie temporarily in the acetabulum.

Each hip should again be examined separately while the opposite thigh is gently fixed by the examiner's other hand. The infant's hip should be flexed to a right angle and the knee more acutely flexed. The examiner should place a thumb as high as possible on the medial aspect of the upper femur while the tips of the middle two fingers grasp the greater trochanter laterally.

The thigh is held lightly in a position of only minimal abduction and then an attempt is made to push the femoral head gently posteriorly and slightly superiorly, while at the same time the examiner's hand is internally rotated through not more than 25°. This is followed by reversing the whole movement. No excessive force is used and only a very limited range of movement employed in the test.

The movement of the head of the femur out and in, or in and out, of the acetabulum produces a jolting or jerking movement, *which can be seen and felt by the examiner. It cannot be heard by an individual with average hearing.* The sensation is like that of a gear lever engaging.

Hips that show excessive movement of the head of the femur within the joint, without being actually dislocatable, are classified as normal.

Ligamentous noise—In at least 10% of infants this examination evokes a noise, click, snap, or grating sensation, but there is no abnormal movement of the femoral head. Such hips should be considered normal and no follow up is required. Because of confusion about its meaning the term "clicking hip" should be abandoned.

Ultrasound in screening

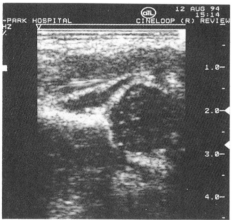

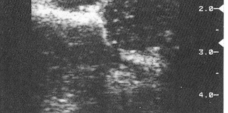

Fem head

Normal hip.

If ultrasound screening is undertaken in every infant before leaving hospital, imaging facilities will be required seven days a week. Twenty per cent of hips may be considered abnormal and the majority will resolve to normal within four weeks.

Selective screening with ultrasound of infants with a clinical hip abnormality or risk factors for congenital dislocated hip (breech delivery, positive family history or foot deformity) reduces the screened population and allows treatment options to be delayed and targeted effectively. A recent study showed that this approach has not reduced the prevalence of late cases of congenital dislocated hip, and it has been suggested that selective ultrasound screening is dependent upon more vigorous clinical screening and careful selection of risk factors.

Ultrasound in diagnosis and management

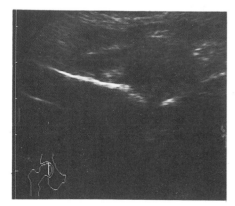

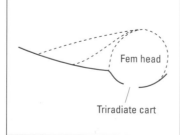

Fem head

Triradiate cart

Abnormal hip (shallow acetabulum).

Delayed ultrasound examination at two weeks in clinically unstable hips will allow treatment to be targeted to those hips that require splintage and thus reduce treatment rates without compromising the results of this treatment.

Weekly ultrasound studies can be used to confirm hip relocation and treatment progress while the infant is in a malleable splint or Pavlik harness. Sonographic evidence of continuing femoral head dislocation, despite splintage, allows treatment to be abandoned and thus the risk of avascular necrosis is reduced. The appearance of the ossific nucleus in the cartilaginous femoral head (usually delayed in congenital dislocated hip) is identified sonographically several weeks before it is visualised radiologically.

Dislocated and dislocatable hip in the newborn

Recommended screening

Babies born after a vertex presentation who have normal hips on clinical examination and do not have any risk factors will continue to receive clinical screening using the neonatal examination and thereafter by their general practitioner in surveillance clinics.

Babies who are judged to be at risk of congenital dislocated hip because they

> **Special risk of congenital dislocated hip**
> - Born in extended breech position
> - Family history of congenital dislocated hip
> - Foot deformity

(a) were born in extended breech position, or
(b) have a family history of congenital dislocated hip, or
(c) have a foot deformity

should have ultrasound in addition to the clinical screening tests. If they are clinically normal and the ultrasound is normal no follow-up is needed. The general practitioner should be sent a standard letter advising that they have been screened by ultrasound but still require follow-up in the surveillance clinic.

If any of the above children have minor abnormalities on the ultrasound scan then they should have a second ultrasound scan six weeks later. Arrangements should be made for them to be reviewed in the paediatric orthopaedic clinic thereafter.

Any child who has a clinically dislocated or dislocatable hip at birth should have an immediate ultrasound and be referred to the next paediatric orthopaedic clinic within a week.

Management of abnormal hips

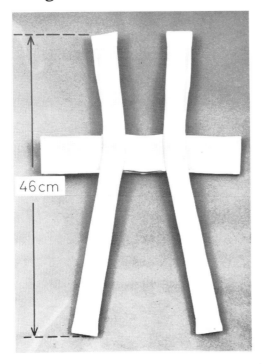

46 cm

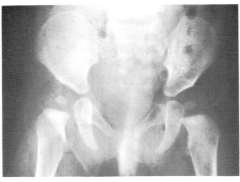

Six months: normal hips.

Apart from cases of irreducible hip dislocation, an infant with a dislocated or dislocatable hip should have a splint applied at about the age of 2 weeks. Further delay may cause poorer results. The Pavlik harness or variants of the von Rosen splint are used. They are made of malleable metal that has been padded and then covered with waterpoof material. The splint acts equally on both hips, keeping both thighs flexed and at an optimum degree of abduction. Unless substitution by a larger splint is required, the splint must remain in position continuously for at least two months if the hip is dislocatable, or for at least three months if it is dislocated at rest. Early consultation with an orthopaedic surgeon, who will continue long-term care, is essential.

Before the splint is first applied, the mother must be told exactly what this treatment entails. She should be encouraged to continue breast feeding, even though this may prove awkward initially. The infant should be placed naked on the splint, which has been fashioned so that the posterior cross bar is grooved to protect the skin over the spine. If the hip is dislocated, the dislocation must first be gently reduced and the thigh held in the abducted position while the splint is carefully applied. Potential pressure points may be protected by inserting pieces of cotton wool or similar material. The mother should be told to replace these when they become wet or soiled without disturbing the splint. The baby's clothes should be put over the splint and not under it.

Once the splint is in place, the infant should be washed, weighed, and examined without the splint being removed. The splint will need scrupulous adjustment at each visit to allow for growth and to ensure that the hip is not being overabducted.

The degree of full abduction in a normal infant diminishes slightly but steadily over the early weeks of life so that the splint should give the comfortable degree of full abduction that is appropriate for the child's age. Failure to adjust progressively for this may cause avascular necrosis of the femoral head. On the other hand, if the degree of thigh abduction is inadequate because the splint is applied too loosely, the hip may remain dislocated. The splint should be checked daily for several days after application and thereafter at intervals of not more than one or two weeks.

Once the splint is finally removed, an anteroposterior radiograph of the hips should be taken with the thighs held parallel, and the infant should be followed up at the ages of 6 and 12 months, at the least.

Late diagnosis

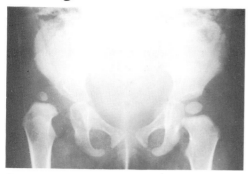

Eighteen months: dislocated hip.

If a dislocated hip is "missed" in the newborn infant the clinical diagnosis is often difficult until, after some weeks, the classical signs of lack of thigh abduction and, in unilateral cases, asymmetry of the lower buttock creases become apparent. Before the age of 4 months an ultrasound study is the most useful aid to diagnosis. Radiologically, once ossification occurs in the upper femoral epiphysis at about the age of 3–4 months a dislocation can be more clearly shown.

WHAT THE FETUS FEELS

The fetal environment is disturbed by sounds, light, and touch, and the fetus responds to these disturbances by moving.

Sound

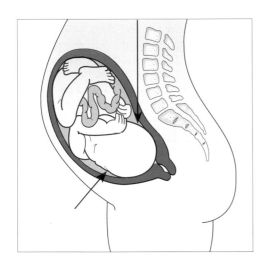

Until the late nineteenth century babies were thought to be born deaf as well as dumb. In fact, the inner ear of the fetus is completely developed by mid-pregnancy, and the fetus responds to a wide variety of sounds.

The fetus is surrounded by a constant very loud noise in the uterus: the rhythmical sound of the uterine blood supply punctuated by the noises of air passing through the mother's intestine. Loud noises from outside the uterus, such as the slamming of a door or loud music, reach the fetus and he reacts to them. The fetus also responds to sounds in frequencies so high or low that they cannot be heard by the human adult ear, which suggests that sensory pathways other than the ear are implicated. Movements of the fetus tend to be inhibited by low frequencies and increased by high frequencies.

Controlled studies in normal pregnancies have demonstrated stimuli such as the application of sound at close quarters does not actually change the heart rate or necessarily awaken fetuses from quiet sleep. However, fetuses definitely do react to vibroacoustic stimulation using an electronic artificial larynx. In normal infants this device can induce excessive fetal movements, a prolonged tachycardia, and abnormal fetal behaviour changes. These effects can last for up to one-and-a-half hours, are quite profound, and occur whatever the behavioural state of the fetus at the time of application. The severity and rapidity of behavioural change has led people to consider that this type of stimulation may be akin to pain and may even be detrimental to the fetus. The use of such stimulation is now no longer recommended.

After birth mothers tend to hold their babies to the left breast. There infants can hear the mother's heartbeat, which provides the same type of rhythm that was present in the uterus and which appears to have a calming effect. Recordings of the adult heartbeat or of the noise in the uterus have a calming effect on infants when they are played to them.

Vision

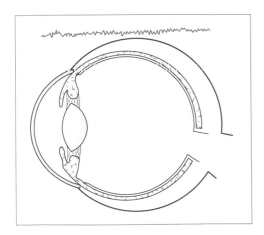

Muscles within the orbit are present very early in pregnancy, and the fetus's eyes move when he changes position and during sleep. In late pregnancy some light penetrates through the uterine wall and amniotic fluid, and fetal activity has been shown to increase in response to bright light, but only in suitably slim mothers.

In preterm infants changes in the electroencephalogram occur in response to light, and the repeated flashing of a light will quieten babies.

Response of touch

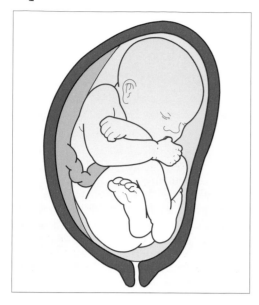

The fetus can touch parts of his body with his hands and feet, and the umbilical cord also touches all parts of his body. Early in pregnancy the fetus tends to move away from objects he touches; later he moves towards them.

Nine weeks after conception the baby is well enough formed for him to bend his fingers round an object in the palm of his hand. In response to a touch on the sole of his foot he will curl his toes or bend his hips and knees to move away from the touching object. At 12 weeks he can close his fingers and thumb, and he will open his mouth in response to pressure applied at the base of the thumb.

At 11 weeks after conception the fetus starts to swallow the surrounding amniotic fluid and to pass it back in his urine. He can also produce complex facial expressions and even smile.

At first when his hands touch his mouth, the fetus turns his head away, though his mouth opens. Later, the fetus may turn his head towards his hands and even put a finger into his open mouth and suck it. This reflex—the rooting reflex—persists after birth. Then it is usually the mother's nipple that touches the baby in this way.

Spontaneous movements

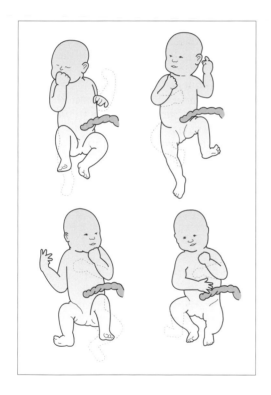

Although fetuses start making spontaneous movements at about seven weeks after conception, mothers do not usually feel their babies moving until about 16 to 21 weeks. The types of movements fetuses make include slow squirmy movements, sharp kicks, and small rhythmic kicks. The squirming tends to increase during pregnancy, while the rhythmic kicks continue at a constant rate from the fifth to the ninth month. The sharp kicks increase up to the seventh month and then diminish due to the relative oligohydramnios.

The fetus's level of activity increases when the mother is under emotional stress. If the stress is prolonged, there is a corresponding increase in the fetus's movements—up to 10 times their normal level. The fetus's activity seems to be increased when the mother is tired.

It is now recognised that fetuses demonstrate clear rest–activity cycle changes, and rapid eye movement sleep can clearly be differentiated from quiet sleep. Disturbances of the rest–activity cycle have now been identified as an early stage of fetal deterioration which is usually associated with abnormal umbilical artery waveforms and precedes qualitative movement changes and reduced fetal body movements.

Towards the end of pregnancy, the fetal chest wall expands and contracts. These movements, which have now been recognised as fetal breathing movements, occur about 70% of the time and are often interrupted by sighs and hiccups. Diminution and cessation of fetal breathing movements as observed by ultrasound are a late sign of fetal asphyxia and may precede fetal death. This, however, is a far from reliable sign, as in some fetuses, acute asphyxia may result in deep gasping movements. Also, immediately before and during labour high levels of maternal prostaglandins inhibit fetal respiratory activity, and in cases of suspected premature labour those infants showing absent fetal breathing movements are more likely to deliver prematurely.

The fetus needs to be heavily sedated by sedating the mother before intrauterine manipulations such as cordocentesis, transfusions, or the insertion of shunts between various fetal cavities and the amniotic fluid. Otherwise the fetus will move away from the needle, which cannot then be inserted. Fetal heart rate and movement increase for a few minutes after tactile stimuli during amniocentesis. The fetus settles down again within a few minutes of the procedure ending.

Changes in heart rate and movement occur that suggest that these stimuli are painful for the fetus. The characteristic fetal response is a severe tachycardia, and excessive fetal movements might well reflect a sudden release of fetal catecholamines and an increase in fetal blood pressure. Certainly it cannot be comfortable for the fetus to have a scalp electrode implanted in the skin, to have blood taken from the scalp, or to suffer the skull compression that may occur even with spontaneous deliveries. It is hardly surprising that infants delivered by difficult forceps extraction act as if they have a severe headache.

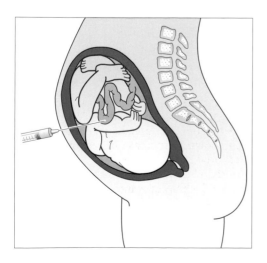

MOTHER–INFANT ATTACHMENT

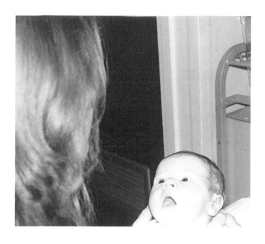

Recent studies have shown that there is no specific sensitive period immediately after delivery that is the only time that attachment can form. Any important effects of separation do not persist beyond days or weeks after reunion. Parents who have read obsolete publications may need reassurance that early separation is not followed by permanent damage to mother–infant relationships. A comparison of preterm and term babies indicated that parents find the behaviour of preterm babies less predictable and more frustrating. Though frequent and sustained contact with a sick or preterm baby may increase the degree of parental anxiety, this anxiety induces a feeling of involvement in the care of their baby.

A biological need

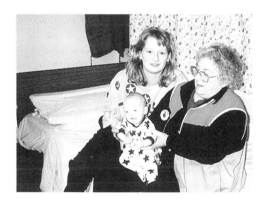

Mothers and infants need a close attachment to give the infant the degree of security necessary for optimal emotional and physical development.

Most mothers have strong maternal feelings, which enable them to achieve a firm bond of affection with their babies without difficulty, even after an initial period of separation. The strength of their maternal feelings probably depends on the quality of mothering they received in infancy.

In contrast, a mother may be unable to achieve this attachment without close contact with her baby, and even then it may take a few days before the baby appears to her to be an individual and her own. Failure to form a normal attachment probably accounts for the higher incidence of "battered babies" among preterm infants and among the infants of mothers who were themselves deprived of maternal care.

Forming an attachment

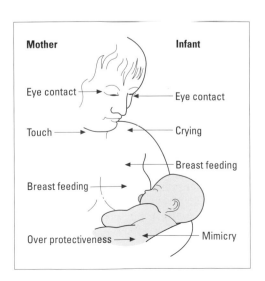

Attachment occurs in five main ways. Firstly, infants can follow the mother's eyes immediately after birth, and this eye-to-eye contact is an important factor.

Secondly, a mother left with her naked infant touches each part of the baby's body with her fingertips.

Thirdly, during the first few days after delivery mothers often appear to overprotect their infants and become overanxious about crying and minor difficulties, such as those of feeding.

Fourthly, even in the first days of life babies mimic the facial expressions of others and can, for example, put out their tongues at them, providing "feedback".

Lastly, physical contact during breast feeding and the presence of the baby next to the mother throughout the entire 24 hours also promote attachment.

Separation

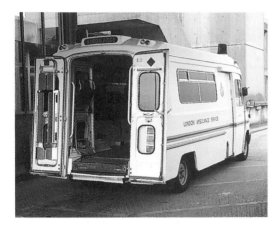

Separation is sometimes unavoidable if, for example, the infant has to be transferred to another unit for surgery or the mother is receiving heavy sedation for hypertension. The mother is equally separated from her child when she is severely depressed, but this may not appear so obvious.

In the past many babies were separated from their mothers for reasons that would not now be acceptable. Owing to doctors' anxiety, infants were cot-nursed after forceps delivery or, if they had prolonged jaundice, admitted to special care units even though they needed no special care. The number of nursing staff available on individual maternity wards will determine whether it is safe for babies to remain with their mothers, but no infant should be separated from his or her mother without good reason.

Part of a postnatal ward may be staffed with midwives who have special experience in nursing babies. This ward is called a transitional ward and allows babies needing tube feeding and other forms of special care to remain with their mothers and avoid the separation resulting from admission to the neonatal unit.

Difficulty in forming attachments

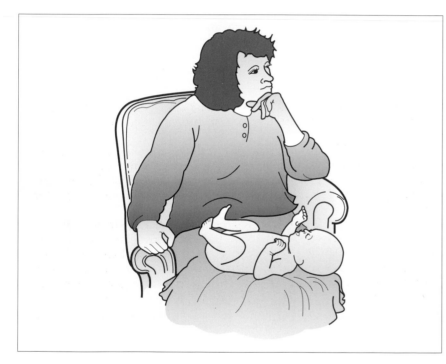

Some aspects of the history may suggest that a mother may have difficulty in forming an attachment to her infant and will need special help from nursing and medical staff. Particularly vulnerable are mothers who had poor maternal care in their own childhood, or who have had a request for an abortion rejected, or unmarried mothers who have not decided whether they want the infant to be adopted. If a previous infant was stillborn or died in the neonatal period or a close relative has recently died, help may also be needed. Special attention should be given to a mother under 17 or over 35 years of age and having her first baby.

When the baby is born, the mother may refuse to handle or feed him or her and be more concerned with her own minor symptoms than the infant's care. She may feel detached, and the infant's problems may appear to her to be more serious than they are. Similar symptoms may be the first indication of a severe depression in the mother, and she may need psychiatric help.

Encouraging attachment

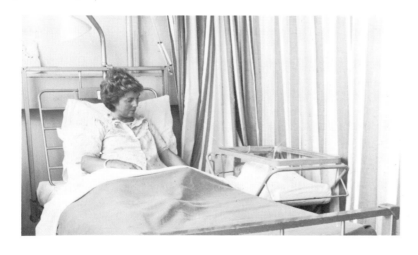

To encourage attachment the principle is to avoid unnecessary separation. Unless infants require special nursing they should be given to their mothers in the labour room, even if an abnormality such as Down's syndrome is present. Newborn infants are able to feed moments after birth even if the mother has received sedation, and the mother should be encouraged to put the baby to her breast if she intends to breast feed. Infants should remain with the mother throughout the 24 hours of the day and be taken out at night only if they continually disturb the other mothers in the room. Breast feeding should be actively encouraged, though this may take time and perseverance by both mothers and nursing

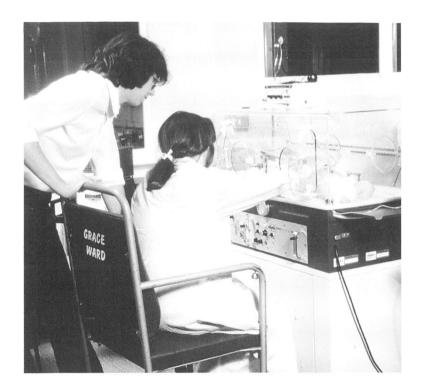

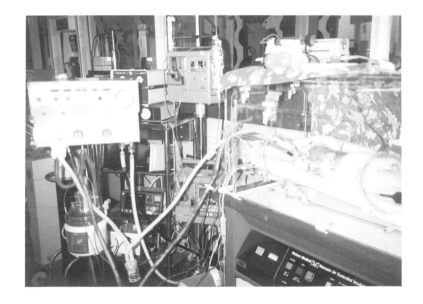

staff. Mothers of preterm infants should be encouraged to express their milk and thus feel that they are actively contributing to the infant's welfare.

In neonatal units the atmosphere should make mothers feel that they are welcome at any time, and they should be encouraged to look at, touch, change, feed, and later breast feed their infants. When the mother is about to visit a very sick infant the reasons for the use of special apparatus should be explained beforehand. A mother can usually visit her infant in the neonatal unit the day after a caesarean section by being wheeled in a chair.

If a mother fails to visit her infant for long periods after she has been discharged, an inquiry should be made whether any remediable reason, such as lack of transport, is responsible.

Before the infant is discharged from the unit the mother should remain with her infant in a room on the unit for at least 24 hours, but longer if possible. This gives her an opportunity to gain confidence in her ability to cope with her baby, who recently appeared to be so fragile and needing expert nursing care to survive.

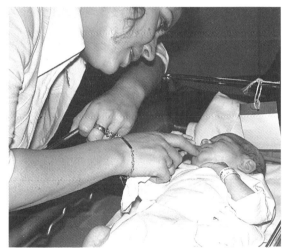

GROWTH AND GROWTH CHARTS

Weight and head circumference

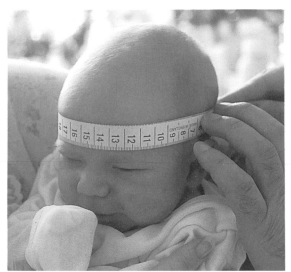

The size of the normal infant at birth is determined mainly by the mother's size. The greatest changes to adjust for other hereditary factors take place during the first three months of life. Although children tend to attain a stature between those of their parents, some children take after one parent, grandparent, or an even more remote member of the family. All these children are perfectly healthy. It may be difficult to distinguish these normal adjustments of growth from disease, especially during the first few months of life. Growth charts are therefore essential for diagnosis during this period and helpful in discussions with parents.

Length (or height) is difficult to measure accurately in a very young baby, and for several years we have used the head circumference as a reference measurement for comparison with the weight. The use of the head circumference in this way is valuable only in the first two years of life. The head circumference is measured round the occipitofrontal circumference (the largest circumference), which should be determined with a disposable paper tape measure. Linen tape measures stretch and produce inaccurate results.

Normal growth and short normal infants

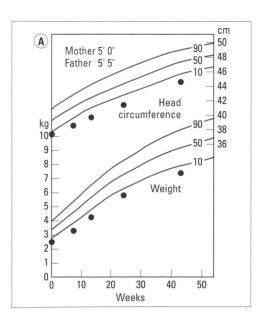

An infant usually has a similar centile at birth for both head circumference and weight. Children of large parents tend to be towards the 90th centile and those of small parents near the 10th centile. Most of these children remain on the same centiles for the rest of their lives. Plotting these measurements on a chart in routine clinics helps to confirm that the child is receiving adequate food and is growing normally.

One of the most common problems in paediatric outpatient clinics is short parents who think that their infant does not eat enough. Plotting growth measurements on a chart from measurements already recorded at the local clinic confirms to the doctor and the parents that the child is normal and that the child's final size will be similar to that of the parents (chart A). Charts are better than cards for recording growth.

Growth and growth charts

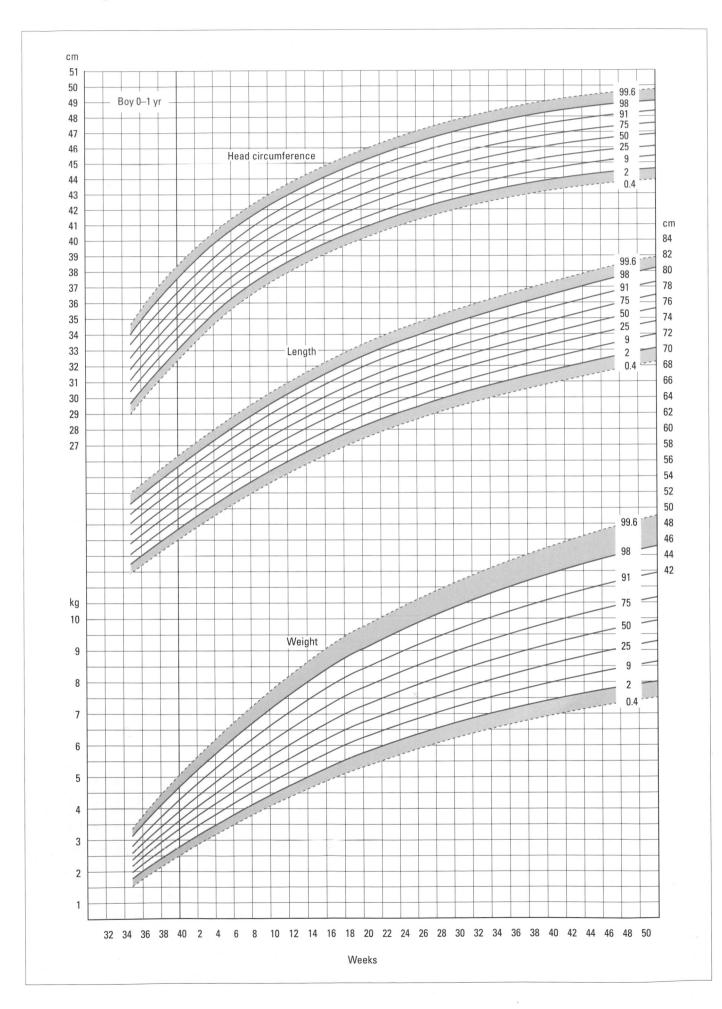

Taking after father or mother

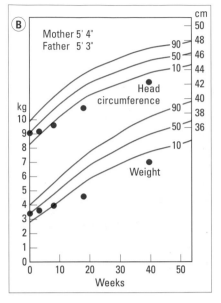

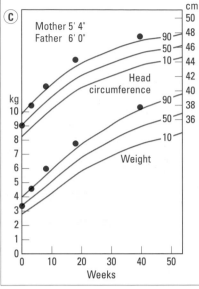

Some children are more similar to one parent than the other in final size. If only their weights are recorded, they may appear to be either failing to thrive if the father is small (chart B) or gaining weight excessively if the father is tall (chart C). If both weight and head circumference are plotted on a chart, the weight centile line and head circumference centile line can be seen to be running in parallel. In other words, the whole of the child's size is approaching that of a particular parent.

Getting fat

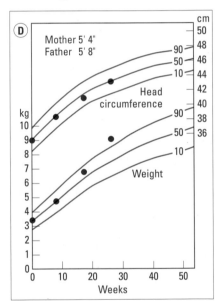

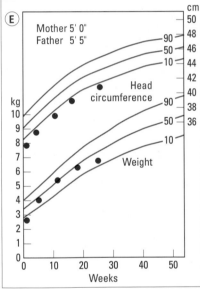

Growth charts give an early warning of obesity. Chart D shows that at the age of 4 months this child's weight centile started deviating upwards although the head circumference centile remained the same. If the mother had been shown the growth chart at the age of 4 months she might have been able to prevent the phenomenon seen at 6 months.

The standard growth charts are based on data collected when the majority of babies were fed with cow's milk preparations. Some normal breast fed babies gain weight rapidly in the first three months and then more slowly during the subsequent three months (chart E). This is a normal growth pattern and is not an indication of obesity.

Poor lactation and failure to thrive

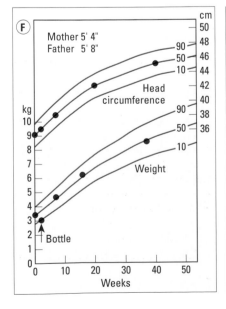

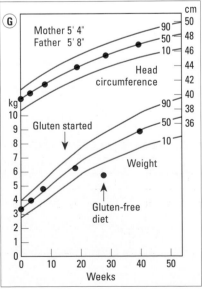

The increasing incidence of breast feeding has resulted in a few infants receiving insufficient milk as a result of their mothers not recognising poor lactation. This can be detected at an early stage by weighing infants regularly, although normal breast fed infants may not regain their birth weights before the age of 2 weeks. The onset of full lactation is extremely variable, and this must be taken into account when considering the adequacy of weight gain (chart F). Plotting the infant's weight on a growth chart is the first investigation required to diagnose whether failure to thrive is present and also to give a presumptive diagnosis of the cause (chart G).

Growth and growth charts

Preterm

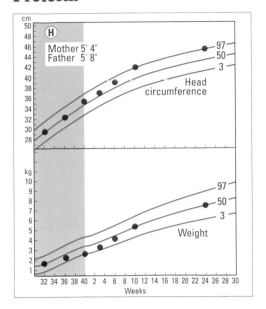

When preterm infants reach home, they may gain weight rapidly, when they will cross the centile lines for both weight and head circumference in parallel (chart H). Preterm infants may have a relatively large head measurement because of the head's discoid shape, but continuing growth on the same centile line shows that the head is normal.

Infant of diabetic mother

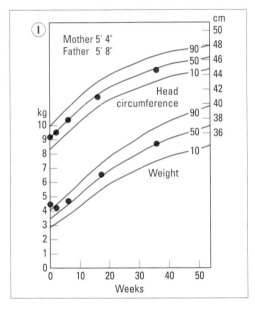

The infant of the diabetic mother may be grossly obese at birth but slims down within a few months of birth (chart I). These infants may not gain any weight at all for the first two months of life and the mother may be accused of starving the infant.

Progressive hydrocephalus

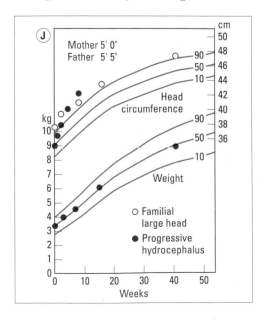

Progressive hydrocephalus can be confirmed by showing a head circumference centile that progressively increases while the weight centile shows no change (chart J). Most of these infants will have associated myelomeningocoele. Hydrocephalus can be confirmed by ultrasound examination of the brain if the anterior fontanelle is still open. This condition must be differentiated from familial large head, where the head circumference centile remains constant and is parallel to the weight centile.

FEEDING AND FEEDING PROBLEMS

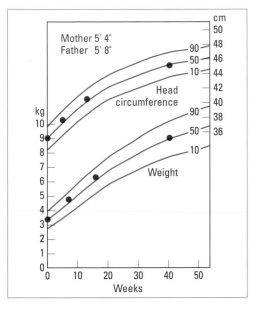

There has been no significant change in the incidence of breast feeding in Great Britain since 1980. In 1990, 63% of mothers breast fed compared with 64% in 1984 and 65% in 1980. There is a steep gradient in the incidence of breast feeding among mothers of first babies from 50% in social class V to 89% in social class I. The incidence of breast feeding among mothers having their first child was 57% for those who left full time education at the age of 16 years or under compared with 93% among mothers who left school at the age of 19. In 1990 one third had stopped breast feeding by 6 weeks. The proportion of breast fed babies receiving additional bottles at 6 weeks has been rising since 1980, when it was 28%, to 34% in 1985 and 39% in 1990.

Full term infants usually regain their birth weight between the seventh and tenth day, and thereafter the infant should gain about 20–40 g/day for the next 100 days. Infants receiving bottled milk ("doorstep" milk) should receive vitamin supplements, particularly vitamin D, until the age of 2 years. Progress on a growth chart is the best guide to ensuring that an infant is receiving the correct amount of milk.

Breast feeding

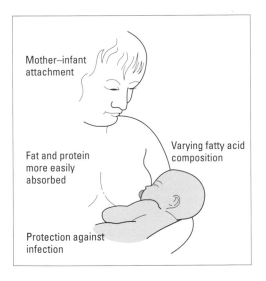

Breast feeding should be encouraged.

Firstly, the fat and protein of human milk are more completely absorbed than those of cows' milk. The composition of human milk varies during a feed, and these subtle changes cannot be mimicked by cows' milk preparations. The significance of these changes is unknown but may be related to the control of intake by appetite.

Secondly, although the fat composition and therefore the fatty acid composition of breast milk vary during a feed, these changes cannot be replaced exactly by cows' milk preparations, and the differences in body composition resulting from these different milks may have a long term effect.

Thirdly, human milk contains antibodies and iron binding protein (lactoferrin) which may protect the infant against infections. Gastroenteritis is rare in breast fed infants.

Breast feeding also plays an important part in mother–infant attachment. If the mother is encouraged during the antenatal period to expect to be able to breast feed her baby and eventually to enjoy it, she is likely to accept early difficulties with patience and understanding. The close contact and intimacy, and often supreme enjoyment, of breast feeding provide the best "feedback" between the baby and the mother. The mother's intimate personal relationship with her baby is something that she has to work out for herself. Many feel insecure and inadequate at first and are only too glad to change to bottle feeding whenever the slightest difficulty arises. The attendant should resist such requests and instead use sympathy, understanding, and skill to encourage the mother to gain confidence in handling her own baby.

Latching to the breast

The sensation of the nipple against the palate stimulates the baby to suck. Placing the baby in the correct position encourages successful feeding and avoids damage to the nipple. The baby's chin must drive into the breast to enable the nipple to reach the palate, so the baby needs to put his head back and up. If the baby's head becomes too flexed, the nipple touches the lower jaw and the tongue and the nose is

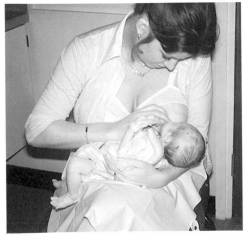

too close to the breast. Helping the chin to thrust forwards and the head to tilt back is hindered by pressure on the back of the head but improved by supporting the baby's back at shoulder level, with the baby facing the mother, chest to chest.

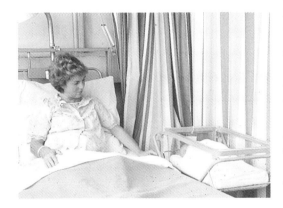

Rooming in

A normal infant is put to the breast for a few minutes at each side either immediately or a few hours after birth. Only a small amount of colostrum is obtained but sucking by the infant stimulates the production of more milk. Some infants are reluctant to take the nipple initially and the mother needs strong reassurance that this is common.

During the first week, and probably later, most of the feed is obtained within four minutes in some babies. Thus the length of time that the baby is on the breast bears little relation to the amount of milk received by the infant. Some infants take a shorter time and others a longer time to take a full feed.

The most satisfactory method of breast feeding is "on demand". Babies commonly feed every two or three hours during the first few weeks and these frequent feeds are a powerful stimulus to lactation. This is the main advantage of rooming in, where the infant's cot is by the side of the mother's bed and she can pick him up and feed him when he cries. Mothers should be encouraged to do this. Infants initially fed on demand usually settle down to a regular schedule after a few weeks. Most breast fed infants feed three hourly rather than four hourly. After the 7th day, if the infant appears to be hungry after a feed or is progressively losing weight test feeding may be considered.

Test feeding

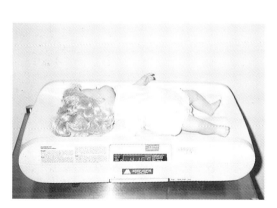

Test feeding should be avoided whenever possible, as it can create anxiety in some mothers. The infant is weighed, without changing the napkin or clothes, before and after each feed during a 24 hour period. If the feed is deficient, putting the baby to the breast more frequently may stimulate increased lactation in the early days or the deficit may be made up with a bottle feed given after feeding from both breasts (complementary feeding). Fortunately, a well nourished full term infant can tolerate a degree of underfeeding without harm for several days.

Complementary feeds are rarely necessary in the first five days, and after this they should be used only when absolutely necessary. The feel of the bottle teat is quite different from that of the nipple, and when the infant is accustomed to one it may be difficult to persuade him to take from the other.

Contraindications to breast feeding

There are few contraindications to breast feeding. Some women have a revulsion to the idea and it would be a mistake to try to persuade them, but psychiatric illness in the mother may be aggravated if the baby is taken off the breast. Severely cracked nipple is a temporary contraindication to feeding from the affected breast, but the milk should be expressed with an electric pump. Feeding should continue from a breast with acute mastitis while the mother is receiving an antibiotic; it should also continue if the nipple is only mildly cracked.

No drugs should be taken by a lactating mother unless there are strong clinical indications. Most drugs that are essential for the mother are secreted in the milk in insignificant amounts, so breast feeding should not be stopped unless there is a special reason. Antibiotics are excreted in minute amounts in the milk but there is the theoretical possibility of sensitising the infant. Warfarin, senna, barbiturates, phenytoin, digoxin, steroids, antacids, and occasional doses of acetylsalicylic acid pass into the milk in unimportant amounts. Kaolin is not absorbed by the mother. Oestrogens in oral contraceptives may reduce lactation, but the progesterone-only pill is an effective contraceptive and has no effect on lactation. A mother receiving carbimazole may continue to breast feed provided that the infant's plasma thyroxine concentration is monitored.

Mothers receiving radioactive antithyroid treatment or cytotoxic drugs should not breast feed. Lithium given to the mother may cause hypotonia, hypothermia, and episodes of cyanosis in a breast fed infant.

Contraindications to breast feeding

- Maternal dislike
- Severely cracked nipple
- *Rarely* drugs

Problems

- Intestinal hurry: *no treatment*

- Cracked nipple: *breast feed or rest*

- Breast engorgement: *expression*

- Gulping: *expression*

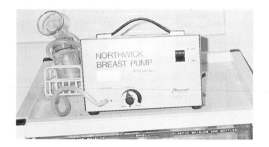

Problems with breast feeding

On the fourth or fifth day, when there is a plentiful supply of breast milk, the infant may take up to eight feeds or more a day. Intestinal hurry and frequent loose green stools are common at this stage. Conversely, some normal breast fed infants pass stools only once a week when they reach the age of a few weeks, and this also requires no treatment.

Cracked nipple is usually due to malplacement of the infant on the nipple so that the whole of the pigmented area is not in the infant's mouth. Pulling the infant off the breast abruptly is another cause. If the nipple is slightly cracked, breast feeding should continue with advice on latching to the breast. If the crack is severe, the infant should be taken off that breast for a day or so and a bland ointment, such as lanolin, placed on the nipple every few hours. A fissure of the nipple occurring after the puerperium is often caused by thrush infection of the baby's mouth and the mother's nipple. It is best treated with miconazole or nystatin gel to both until four days after it appears to be clear.

In acute mastatis there is fever, pain, flushing, and induration in one breast and enlarged axillary lymph nodes. Flucloxacillin or erythromycin is given to the mother for at least a week and feeding continues from both breasts. Fluctuation in the indurated area indicates that an abscess is present and the need for surgical incision and suppression of lactation with bromocryptine.

Feeding on demand usually prevents maternal breast engorgement, which can occur towards the end of the first week of the baby's life. This is easily alleviated by expression after feeding, preferably with an electric pump. If engorgement has already occurred the help of an experienced midwife is necessary.

During the first feed of the morning milk may spurt quickly from the breast and a ravenous infant may swallow excessive air, which may be regurgitated later with milk. This is often accompanied by severe crying. It can be alleviated by manual expression of the first 30 ml of milk, which can be given to the infant later if necessary.

Bottle feeding

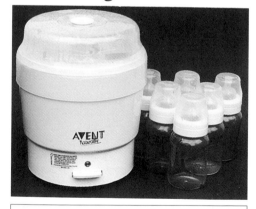

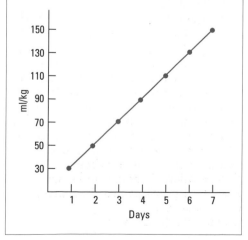

All the cows' milk preparations available in Britain have sodium and protein concentrations similar to those of human milk. Unlike the older cows' milk preparations, they are less likely to be associated with hypernatraemia, hypocalcaemia, and obesity. The powder should be measured accurately, avoiding heaped or packed scoops. The instructions on each packet must be followed. Some preparations are available in liquid form and although heavier parcels need to be carried from the clinic, the milk can be measured out more accurately. Ready to feed bottles are used in most obstetric units.

If feeds are made up for a 24 hour period they should be stored in the refrigerator. Bottles can be sterilised in dilute hypochlorite solution, but processing in an autoclave is the best method in hospitals. Other methods include steam or a special microwave oven kit. Teats should be well washed before sterilisation.

The size of the hole in the teat should allow individual drops of milk to follow each other quickly when the bottle is inverted, and this should be checked each week.

"On demand" feeding

Feeds are usually given "on demand" or three or four hourly. Most infants need to be fed every three hours. The milk must not be made up to a stronger concentration than that recommended on the packet. Few babies can manage without a night feed for the first few months.

A normal full term infant receives 30 ml of milk per kg body weight during the first day of feeding by bottle. Feeds should be increased by 20 ml/kg each day until a maximum of 150 ml/kg is reached on the seventh day of feeding. Underfeeding causes small amounts of green mucus to be passed frequently, but this is more likely to be found with breast fed than with bottle fed infants.

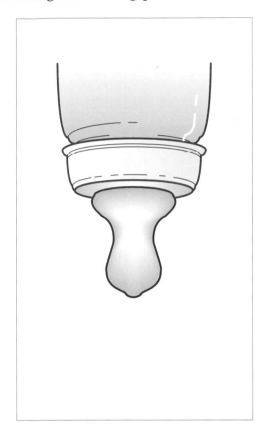

Problems with bottle feeding

If the hole in the teat is too small the infant may swallow excessive air during the feed and regurgitate it later with milk, accompanied by bouts of crying. It is valuable to observe the rate at which the drops of milk are formed when the infant's bottle is inverted. The drops should follow each other quickly but there should not be a continuous stream. If the hole is too small it may be made larger with a hot needle. If the hole is too large, infants may swallow excessive air as they gulp to avoid choking.

By taking a careful history it is usually possible to determine the likely cause of any symptoms. If growth is poor, infants need more frequent or larger feeds. If the weather is hot and infants are not receiving extra water, they may be thirsty and should have additional water. Mothers tend to use gripe water as a panacea, not realising that it contains bicarbonbate, which produces carbon dioxide in the stomach.

Reluctance to feed

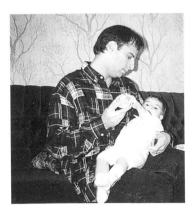

In an infant who has fed normally before, reluctance to feed may be a dangerous symptom. It may be due to any severe disease, such as congenital heart disease or a lower respiratory tract infection. On the other hand, when an infant has a mild upper respiratory tract infection the nose may become blocked with mucus, making it difficult for the baby to feed. Thrush produces white plaques on the buccal mucosa and tongue, which become sore. It can be treated by a five-day course of oral nystatin drops or miconazole oral gel, 1 ml twice a day.

FAILURE TO THRIVE

Is the weight gain normal?
If not, what is the cause?

Mothers become anxious if their infants do not gain weight at the rate that is expected. The majority of these babies are perfectly healthy but the expectations are too high. Initially, it is essential to determine whether the baby is gaining weight normally. If weight gain is abnormal, failure to thrive is present and a cause should be sought. Some of the material in this chapter is also found in "Growth and growth charts".

Normal weight gain

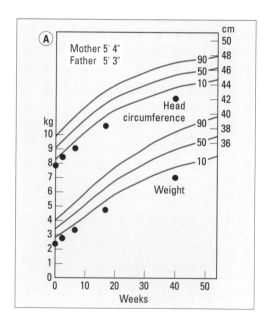

Small parents

An infant usually has a similar centile at birth for both head circumference and weight. Children of large parents tend to be towards the 90th centile and those of small parents near the 10th centile. Most of these children remain on the same centiles for the rest of their lives. Plotting these measurements on a chart helps to confirm that children are receiving adequate food and are growing normally. A common problem is the infant of short parents who consider that their child does not eat enough. Plotting growth measurements on a chart from measurements already recorded at the local clinic confirms to the doctor and the parents that the child is normal and that his or her final size will be similar to that of the parents. Charts are better than lists of measurements for seeing the trends in growth.

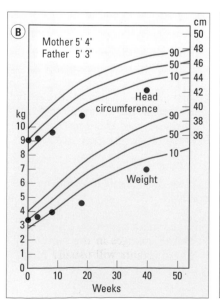

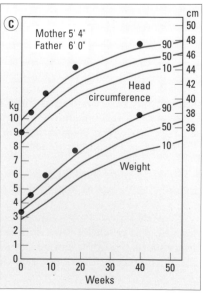

Taking after father or mother

Some children are more similar to one parent than the other in final size. If only their weight is recorded they may appear to be either failing to thrive if the father is small (chart B) or gain in weight excessively if the father is tall (chart C). If both weight and head circumference are plotted on a chart, the weight centile line and head circumference centile line can be seen to be running in parallel. In other words, the whole of the child's size is approaching that of a particular parent.

Failure to thrive

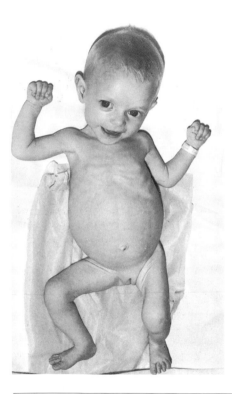

Low birth weight

Infants who are of low birth weight may have been born early (preterm) or have experienced intrauterine malnutrition or both. Although some of them have a period of "catch up" growth during the first few months of life, others remain below the 10th centile for the whole of their lives. This is considered to be related to the intrauterine malnutrition (see chart D).

Physical causes of failure to thrive

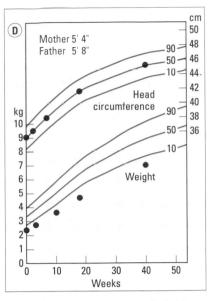

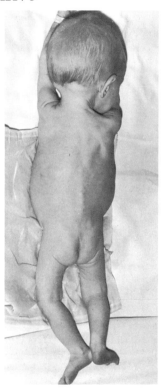

A progressive fall in the weight centile with a constant head circumference centile is the best confirmation of failure to thrive. Measurements on a single occasion may show a weight centile that is below the head circumference and length centile, but these findings may be present in a normal baby whose family has a body shape that is slightly different from the majority. The plotting of serial measurements on a growth chart before starting to take a history often shortens that process.

Deficient intake of food or the excessive loss from malabsorption or metabolic disease cause failure to thrive. Psychiatric and social problems, which are the predominant factor in the majority of the infants with failure to thrive in this country, probably reduce the food intake.

A detailed history is taken, paying particular attention to the family history, birth, feeding, and maternal anxieties. Details of any vomiting, diarrhoea, or abdominal distension are noted. The complete examination includes an assessment of developmental age and evidence of wasting, particularly of the inner aspects of the thighs and buttocks.

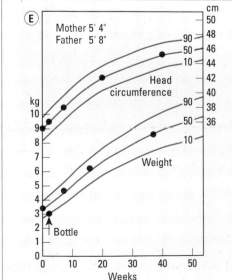

Deficient intake

Poor lactation—The high incidence of breast feeding in some areas has resulted in a few infants receiving insufficient milk as a result of their mothers' not recognising poor lactation. This can be detected at an early stage by weighing infants regularly, although normal breast fed infants may not regain their birth weights before the age of 2 weeks. The onset of full lactation is extremely variable, and this must be taken into account when considering the adequacy of weight gain (see "Feeding and feeding problems").

Problems with bottle feeding—Poor tuition may result in deficient milk intake (see "Feeding and feeding problems").

Cerebral palsy—Infants with cerebral palsy may present with slow feeding and resulting poor milk intake before changes in the motor function in the limbs can be detected. These infants will usually have some evidence of developmental delay.

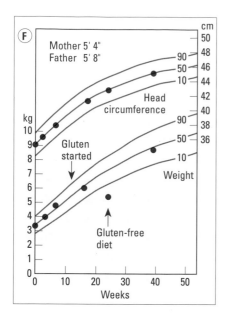

Congenital heart disease—There may be deficient milk intake due to slow feeding and there is also a high metabolic rate. Central cyanosis, a murmur, or both are usually present.

Urinary infection—A clean catch urine specimen examined promptly in the laboratory is essential for this diagnosis.

Excessive loss

Gastro-oesophageal reflux—Persistent vomiting from birth may result in failure to thrive if the infant does not take in additional milk to compensate for the loss (see page 53).

Congenital pyloric stenosis—This condition may present any time until the age of 2 months. It should be considered in any baby less than that age who vomits persistently (see page 52).

Malabsorption—In this country the main causes of malabsorption are cows' milk protein intolerance, cystic fibrosis, and coeliac disease. These conditions all cause loose stools that are more frequent than normal but this may not be recognised by a mother with a first child. A detailed history of bowel function should be taken and personal examination of the stool may be helpful.

Diabetes mellitus—This can be excluded by a negative multistix test for glucose in the urine.

Psychiatric and social factors of failure to thrive

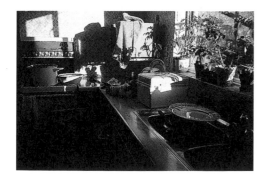

A physical cause for failure to thrive may be present in a family with psychiatric and social problems and therefore a physical cause must be excluded for all infants. The exclusion of a physical cause is often helpful in persuading the parents to accept that psychiatric or social factors are the main reason for the problem. Features in the history that may suggest this possibility include maternal depression, marital discord, or a disorganised household. Maternal food preferences may result in the exclusion of certain foods, such as cows' milk, from the diet without reason and without adequate supervision, and may result in a deficient energy intake.

There are more subtle ways in which maternal emotional factors may affect the infant. The mother may be depressed and tense, and this anxiety is transmitted to the child, who does not feed. The mother then reacts by removing the food. In other families the child may be intrinsically less responsive than the average child to food and this may affect the mother's response to the child at mealtimes. In both these examples the amount of food taken by the child falls to a plateau where the infant appears to be satisfied with the amount given. Another possibility is that the mother keeps to a diet herself as she perceives that she is overweight and also gives a diet to the infant in a similar way.

Some infants are deliberately underfed as part of child abuse. Normal weight gain occurs when fostering has been carried out.

Effective management of infants with this diagnosis requires a team approach involving a health visitor, the family doctor, a child psychiatrist, and paediatrician.

Investigations

Specific investigations are indicated by the history and examination given above, but if there are no pointers to the diagnosis the following investigations are performed: Multistix urine test for glucose, full blood count, sweat test, urine microscopy and culture, and plasma creatinine.

JAUNDICE IN THE NEWBORN

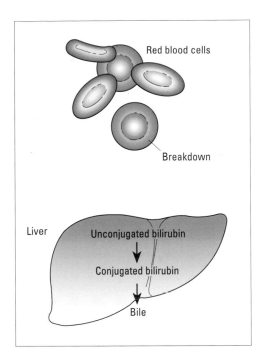

Jaundice is a yellow colour of the skin caused by a high concentration of bilirubin. Very severe jaundice may damage the cells of the basal ganglia and brain stem. This damage is produced by the fat soluble unconjugated bilirubin. If jaundice is severe, high bilirubin levels may result in deafness, cerebral palsy, or death.

Neonatal jaundice is due to an increased bilirubin load with a transient inefficiency of hepatic excretion resulting from decreased activity of glucuronyl transferase in the liver. There are additional factors. Some of the conjugated bilirubin excreted in the bile is normally deconjugated in the small intestine and reabsorption is enhanced by the slower gut transit in the starved new born. Bilirubin is absorbed from meconium and there is no intestinal flora to degrade bilirubin to urobilinogen.

Common causes of jaundice in the newborn

Cause	Onset
Red cell incompatability	Within 24 hours of birth
Physiological jaundice	After 24 hours
Septicaemia	Usually after fourth day

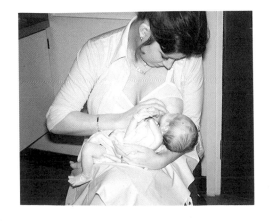

Common causes of jaundice include hepatic immaturity, red cell incompatibility, infection, and breast feeding.

Jaundice due to hepatic immaturity, or "physiological" jaundice, is common both in preterm and in full-term babies. A temporary deficiency of glucuronyl transferase enzymes reduces the rate of conjugation of bilirubin, with a consequent retention of unconjugated bilirubin. In full-term infants the jaundice always appears after the first 24 hours of life and reaches a peak on the fourth or fifth day. In preterm infants it usually begins 48 hours after birth and may last up to two weeks.

In babies with red cell incompatibility jaundice appears within 24 hours of birth. The main causes are: (a) incompatible rhesus grouping, and (b) incompatible ABO grouping; the mother's blood is usually group O and the infant's group A or, less commonly, group B.

The common infective causes of jaundice are septicaemia and urinary tract infection. Septicaemia is especially likely to be present if the jaundice appears after the fourth day of life, but it is a possibility in any infant who seems ill. In urinary tract infections the jaundice is of hepatic origin.

In about 2·5% of infants who are breast fed the serum bilirubin rises to levels between 260 and 360 μmol/l in the second or third week of life. These infants have no symptoms. If breast feeding continues the level remains constant for three or four weeks and falls to normal levels at 4–16 weeks. An abnormal progesterone has been shown in the milk of some of the mothers.

Rare causes of jaundice in the newborn

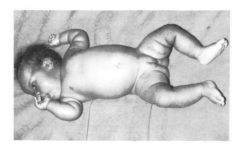

- Hypothyroidism
- Galactosaemia
- Viral hepatitis
- Atresia of bile ducts
- Glucose-6-phosphate dehydrogenase deficiency

Rare causes of jaundice include hypothyroidism, galactosaemia, viral hepatitis, and atresia of the bile ducts. These cause prolonged jaundice lasting more than 10 days. Glucose-6-phosphate dehydrogenase deficiency is another cause of prolonged jaundice, but it can also produce a clinical picture similar to blood group incompatibility.

In hypothyroidism physiological jaundice is prolonged, the plasma thyroxine (T4) concentration is reduced, and the thyroid stimulating hormone (TSH) concentration is increased.

In infants with viral hepatitis, which is usually due to intrauterine infection, the stools are pale, the urine dark owing to bile, and there is a high level of conjugated bilirubin in the plasma.

It is difficult to differentiate between hepatitis and atresia of the bile ducts clinically, and they may represent the two ends of a range of disease. If jaundice persists more than 10 days, the advice of a paediatrician should be sought.

In galactosaemia the urine gives a positive result on testing for reducing substances, but the test for glucose may be negative. The infant needs to be referred to a paediatrician immediately for special investigations.

Glucose-6-phosphate dehydrogenase deficiency occurs in infants of Mediterranean, African, or Chinese stock. This hereditary red cell enzyme defect is found in babies with haemolytic episodes that often occur without the usual precipitating factors of drugs or infection. The enzyme is necessary for maintaining the stability of the red-cell membrane.

Management of jaundice starting in the first 24 hours

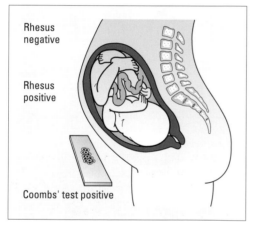

Rhesus incompatibility.

Onset within first 24 hours—whatever the level

- Serum bilirubin—both conjugated and unconjugated
- Full blood count and blood film
- Blood group
- Coombs' test

If jaundice appears within 24 hours of birth it must be considered to be due to blood group incompatibility, with a high risk of cerebral palsy, until proved otherwise. Most rhesus problems should be anticipated before the neonatal period. Urgent exchange transfusion may be indicated in infants severely affected by haemolytic disease of the newborn, and it is advisable for the infant to be admitted to hospital immediately for investigation. If the mother is rhesus negative, the infant rhesus positive, and the Coombs test positive, jaundice is due to rhesus incompatibility. The plasma bilirubin concentration should be measured every five to eight hours and the results plotted on a special chart (see page 48). Once the second estimation has been performed the maximum concentration can be predicted, as the rate of increase is linear. When the serial concentrations fall below the printed line, the infant is unlikely to need any treatment.

Management of jaundice starting after the first 24 hours

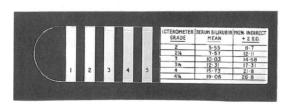

The possibility of septicaemia or urinary tract infection should be considered in any ill baby who develops jaundice after the first 24 hours of life. If there is any doubt about when the jaundice first appeared, the possibility of blood group incompatibility should be investigated.

When a doctor visits the infant at home a guide to the plasma bilirubin concentration can be provided by the dermal icterometer. This is a piece of transparent perspex with yellow lines of various shades that

Jaundice in the newborn

Onset after 24 hours but serum bilirubin >300 μmol/l

- Serum bilirubin—conjugated and unconjugated
- Full blood count and white count differential
- Blood group
- Coombs' test
- Blood culture
- Urine culture (for asymptomatic infection)
- Glucose-6-phosphate dehydrogenase levels in the appropriate racial groups

correspond to plasma bilirubin concentrations. It should be compressed gently on the infant's nose to indicate the approximate plasma bilirubin concentrations. The dermal icterometer is not accurate in artificial light, when bilirubin values are rising rapidly, or when phototherapy has been given. In infants with pigmented skin the dermal icterometer should be compressed against the gums, not the nose.

In full-term infants if the dermal icterometer suggests that the plasma bilirubin concentration is about 250 μmol/l or the result lies above the line on the chart the infant should be tranferred to hospital immediately. If the plasma bilirubin level is very high, urgent exchange transfusion or phototherapy may be needed.

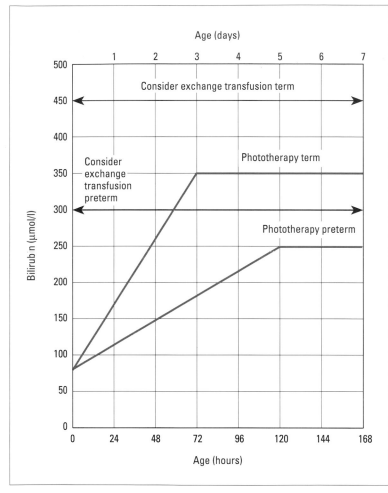

Bilirubin chart
400 μmol/l = 23·4 mg/100 ml
300 μmol/l = 17·5 mg/100 ml
200 μmol/l = 11·7 mg/100 ml
100 μmol/l = 5·8 mg/100 ml
17·1 μmol/l = 1·0 mg/100 ml

In neonatal units there is usually a ward bilirubinometer that measures plasma bilirubin concentrations within a few minutes, using a small specimen of blood obtained by heel prick. If two estimations fall below the line on the chart, treatment will probably not be needed. Those with values above the line may need exposure to light under a phototherapy unit. Phototherapy produces geometric stereoisomers of bilirubin, which have no known long-term deleterious effect on the infant. The infant's eyes are shielded with eye pads held in place with Micropore tape, but the mother should have the procedure explained first. Although phototherapy units have a shield to reduce transfer of heat from the lamp to the infant, monitoring of the temperature of the infant is essential. Extra fluids may be needed to compensate for the additional evaporative loss and this can be given as plain water to breast fed infants or additional milk to bottle fed babies. Oral fluid decreases the gut transit time and improves the excretion of bilirubin and the associated compounds. The indications for phototherapy are controversial but many units give phototherapy if the plasma bilirubin level is above the line on the chart. Despite phototherapy, an exchange transfusion may still be needed, but the critical level varies with the unit and the gestational age of the infant. Exchange transfusion should be considered if the plasma bilirubin level exceeds 450 μmol/l in a full term infant and 300 μmol/l in a preterm infant. Some units start treatment at lower levels of bilirubin in sick infants.

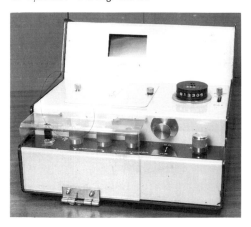

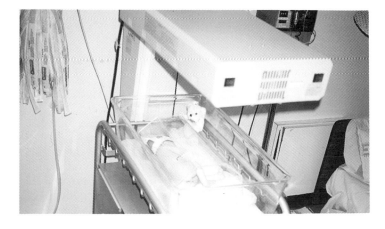

Prolonged jaundice

Prolonged jaundice > 14 days

- Serum bilirubin—conjugated and unconjugated
- Full blood count
- Thyroid function tests
- Liver enzymes
- Glucose-6-phosphate dehydrogenase if appropriate
- Urine culture
- Urine for reducing substances (for galactosaemia)
- Urine for presence of bilirubin which reflects a high conjugated bilirubin (on a Labstix).

If jaundice persists longer than 14 days in a full-term infant, blood should be taken for plasma thyroxine and thyroid stimulating hormone estimations and a specimen of urine collected to measure reducing substances and glucose. The urine should be examined in the laboratory for the presence of infection. If the parents are of Mediterranean, African, or Chinese origin, the screening test for red cell glucose-6-phosphate dehydrogenase should also be performed.

Pale stools and a plasma conjugated bilirubin level greater than 30 μmol/l suggest the possibility of hepatitis or atresia of the bile ducts, and the advice of a paediatrician is needed.

If there is a suspicion that the jaundice is related to breast feeding, the other conditions causing jaundice should be excluded and the mother advised to continue breast feeding. If the plasma bilirubin concentration is rising rapidly and breast feeding is stopped for 48 hours, the infant's plasma bilirubin concentration will fall abruptly and will not usually rise on return to breast feeding. Although the mother can continue lactation by expressing her milk during this diagnostic test there is a risk that breast feeding will not be resumed.

VOMITING

Vomiting in the newborn: types of vomit

- Frothy
- Bile stained
- Blood stained
- Milk

Vomiting is the forceful expulsion of gastric contents through the mouth. Mothers often confuse vomiting with mild regurgitation, which is the effortless bringing up of small amounts of milk during and between feeds, usually accompanied by air. If the milk dribbles down the chest it is likely to be regurgitation. Babies often bring up small amounts of milk with air, and this is of no importance. Recurrent vomiting may be a sign of lethal disease, but a careful history and examination enable a diagnosis to be made with the minimum of special investigations.

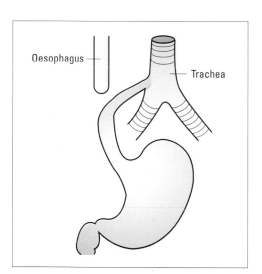

Frothy mucoid vomit

Oesophageal atresia with tracheo-oesophageal fistula may present with vomiting, coughing, and cyanosis when the infant begins the first feed. Many of these infants drool frothy material continuously rather than vomit. Vomiting of *frothy* mucoid material may be the only definite observation, but the condition should be suspected in any baby who has *any* symptoms during the first feed. As the fluid expelled is not gastric contents, vomiting is not an accurate description but this is the term often used.

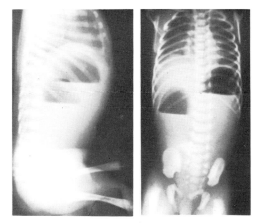

Erect lateral (left) and antero-posterior (right) radiographs to show fluid levels.

Bile stained vomit

The vomit in infants with intestinal obstruction is usually yellow, due to bile staining, but occasionally it consists only of milk. The cause may be atresia, stenosis, or volvulus of the small gut, necrotising enterocolitis, or congenital intestinal aganglionosis (Hirschsprung's disease) of the large gut. Abdominal distension is usually present and there may be visible peristalsis. A plain radiograph should be taken in the erect position immediately. An alternative is a radiograph in the supine position and, in addition, a lateral view with the baby lying on his or her back and a horizontal x-ray beam. They often show fluid levels, dilated loops of gut proximal to the obstruction, and the absence of gas shadows distally. Ideally, every infant who vomits bile should be seen by a surgeon within an hour.

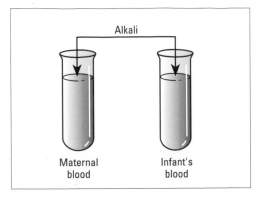

Maternal blood — Infant's blood
Alkali

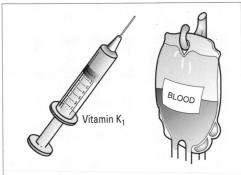

Vitamin K₁ — BLOOD

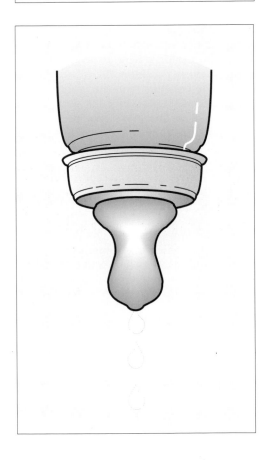

Bloodstained vomit

Bloodstained vomit may be caused by trauma from a feeding tube, swallowed maternal blood, or, most seriously, haemorrhagic disease of the newborn. Trauma caused by a feeding tube may produce a few specks of blood in the vomit. Maternal blood may be swallowed before delivery after premature separation of the placenta or after delivery as the result of bleeding from a cracked nipple. Maternal haemoglobin in the vomit can be recognised in the laboratory.

Haemorrhagic disease of the newborn begins between the second and fourth days of life in the early type, or in the third or fourth week in the late type. The first symptom may be haematemesis or melaena, and the bleeding can be profuse. An immediate dose of 1 mg vitamin K_1 should be given intramuscularly and a transfusion of fresh blood given urgently if bleeding has been severe or persists after vitamin K treatment.

Milk

Vomiting of milk may be caused by infections, feeding problems, necrotising enterocolitis, intracranial haemorrhage, or drugs.

Gastroenteritis, urinary tract infection, septicaemia, and meningitis may all be associated with vomiting. A ravenous infant may swallow excessive air at the beginning of the feed, and if not properly "winded", may later regurgitate milk with air. Larger feeds, more frequent feeds, or a larger hole in the teat is needed.

Necrotising enterocolitis occurs in epidemics in neonatal baby units. Lethargy and refusal of feeds are followed by vomiting and abdominal distension. In the majority of the infants there is melaena. Predisposing factors are prematurity, perinatal hypoxia, hypotension, umbilical vessel catheterisation, and prolonged rupture of the membranes. Embolism or thrombosis of mesenteric vessels is followed by ischaemic changes, which vary from mucosal ulceration to complete necrosis of the gut wall. Bacteria invade the necrotic tissue and healing is followed by scarring and sometimes a stricture. Despite optimal treatment there is a 25% mortality rate and early advice from a paediatric surgeon is advisable.

Raised intracranial pressure due to intracranial haemorrhage may cause vomiting of milk, as may several drugs, especially digoxin.

Vomiting from the first week to the first year: causes

- ● **Feeding problems**
- ● **Infections**
  Urinary tract infection
  Septicaemia
  Meningitis

As in the newborn, vomiting in infants older than 1 week may be a symptom of a feeding problem or an infection such as urinary tract infection, otitis media, gastroenteritis, septicaemia, or meningitis (see page 80).

If no cause of the vomiting is found and the symptoms are mild, urine should be collected for microscopy and culture, and should be examined for protein, bile, and reducing substances.

Vomiting

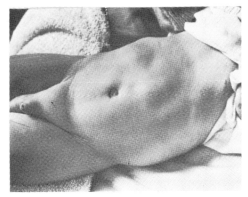

Pyloric stenosis.

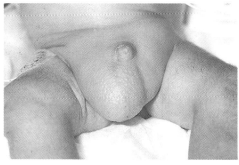

Inguinal hernia.

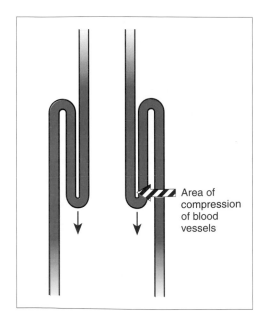

Area of compression of blood vessels

Pyloric stenosis

Pyloric stenosis must be considered in every infant less than 3 months of age who vomits. Rarely the vomiting may occur in the first week of life, but it usually begins in the second or third week, though there may be a delay before the infant is seen by a doctor. Usually the vomit is produced forcefully and reaches some distance from the infant. The infant often accepts another feed immediately after vomiting. Stools are infrequent. If the symptoms have been present for more than a few days, there will be a loss of weight due to dehydration and loss of subcutaneous fat. Scanty urine is associated with dehydration.

The essential diagnostic sign is the presence of a pyloric mass palpated during a test feed. Constant practice is needed to appreciate a pyloric mass. Even if no pyloric mass is felt during the first test feed, if the diagnosis of pyloric stenosis is probable the infant should be admitted for rehydration and the examination repeated. Preliminary aspiration and measurement of gastric contents is helpful, particularly if no feed has been given during the preceding four hours. Metabolic alkalosis strongly suggests the diagnosis.

In a small proportion of infants the diagnosis of pyloric stenosis is suspected clinically but no pyloric mass is palpable during a test feed. The diagnosis may be confirmed, preferably by an ultrasound study. A barium study is needed rarely.

Intestinal obstruction

Infants who vomit yellow bile are likely to have intestinal obstruction. They should be admitted immediately and seen by a surgeon within an hour. Abdominal distension is often present and peristalsis may be visible. Duodenal stenosis usually presents during the first few days of life but malrotation of the gut with associated volvulus may produce symptoms at any time during childhood.

An inguinal hernia is more likely to incarcerate in the early months of life than later. Incarceration should be suspected if the hernia is tender or is not reduced easily; immediate surgery is required. The risk of obstruction is always present and early surgical treatment is advisable in every baby with an inguinal hernia. The baby must remain in the ward until the operation is performed.

An intussusception is a partial or complete intestinal obstruction due to invagination of a portion of the gut into a more distal portion. It may occur at any age, although the maximum incidence is at 3–11 months. An intussusception may be easily diagnosed in a child who has all the typical features, but these children are not common. The distinctive feature is the periodicity of the attacks, which may consist of severe screaming, drawing up of the legs, and severe pallor. Some episodes consist of pallor alone. The attack lasts a few minutes and may recur about 20 minutes later, though attacks may be more frequent. There may be vomiting and one or two loose stools may be passed initially, suggesting acute gastroenteritis. Bloodstained mucus may be passed rectally or shown by rectal examination. But some patients pass no blood rectally. Between attacks the infant appears normal and may have no abnormal signs apart from a palpable mass.

It is difficult to examine the abdomen during an attack because the child cries continuously, but between attacks a mass, most commonly over the right upper quadrant, can be felt in 70% of children.

If surgical shock is present, then rapid resuscitation should be carried out and intravenous fluids, including blood, given. Plain radiographs of the abdomen may show evidence of intestinal obstruction or a density in the area of the lesion. Ultrasound shows a doughnut configuration with hypoechogenic rims and a dense central echogenic core. An urgent surgical opinion should be obtained. If the symptoms have been present for less than 48 hours, and there are no signs of intestinal perforation, a barium enema should be given urgently while the surgeon remains nearby. In over 75% of cases it is possible to reduce the intussusception by the hydrostatic pressure of the barium. If the intussusception is not reduced, then immediate laparotomy is needed to reduce the lesion manually or to perform an intestinal resection. In about 6% of cases there is a persisting mechanical cause of the intussusception and this will not be detected by the barium enema.

Gastro-oesophageal reflux

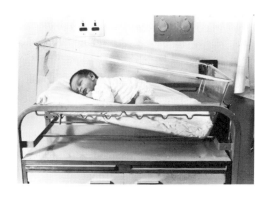

Vomiting due to gastro-oesophageal reflux starts during the first week of life and the vomitus may be blood stained. Aspiration into the lungs may cause recurrent bronchospasm and severe vomiting may cause failure to thrive, dysphagia, or stricture formation. During the first year the lower oesophageal sphincter pressure increases and oesophageal mobility becomes more organised. These factors reduce the regurgitation of gastric contents into the oesophagus when the intra-abdominal pressure rises, for example during crying.

The diagnosis is confirmed by 24 hour pH monitoring of the lower oesophagus. A probe the size of a naso-gastric tube is placed just above the gastro-oesophageal sphincter. The pH recording is analysed by computer. Barium swallow examination is often negative despite typical symptoms.

Vomiting usually resolves by the age of 1 year without specific treatment. If symptoms are severe, the feeds can be thickened with instant Carobel and the infant may be nursed with his head higher than his feet on his side. If the vomiting is persistent and severe, a paediatrician may prescribe cisapride, which alters oesophageal motility, and cimetidine, which reduces acid production by the stomach.

Whooping cough

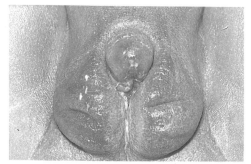

Catarrhal phase	Paroxysmal phase	Convalescent phase
Short dry cough at night	Vomiting and whooping Bouts of 10–20 coughs at day and night	Coughing

1 — Weeks → 8

Vomiting may be so severe in infants with whooping cough that the mother is more worried by the vomiting than the cough. During the first five days of the illness (catarrhal phase) there is a short, dry nocturnal cough. Later, bouts of 10 to 20 short coughs occur day and night. The cough is dry and each cough is on the same high note or goes up in a musical scale. The long attack of coughing is followed by a sharp indrawing of breath, which causes the whoop. Some children with proved pertussis infection never develop the whoop. Feeding often provokes a spasm of coughing and this may culminate in vomiting. Afterwards there is a short refractory period during which the baby can be fed again without provoking more coughing. In uncomplicated cases there are no abnormal signs in the respiratory system.

Adrenogenital syndrome

Adrenogenital syndrome.

The adrenogenital syndrome (salt losing type) commonly presents with vomiting as the only symptom in boys. The diagnosis is easier in girls, as virilisation of the external genitalia will have been noticed at birth. Symptoms usually begin between the seventh and tenth days, and may be fatal within a few days if extra salt and salt-retaining adrenocorticosteroids are not given. Intravenous fluids are essential. The diagnosis is confirmed by raised plasma 17 OH-progesterone concentrations, high plasma potassium, and low plasma sodium concentrations. The plasma electrolyte concentrations are normal at birth, and pronounced changes may occur suddenly.

DIARRHOEA

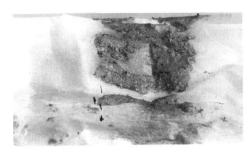

Loose stool.

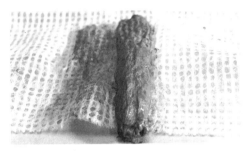

Normal stool.

Diarrhoea is the passage of loose stools more often than would be expected from the diet and age of the infant. It indicates a change in bowel habit. A stool should be examined personally. A rectal examination or the passage of a rectal thermometer is often followed by a fresh stool, which can be examined. When diarrhoea is severe, the stools may be mistaken for urine. When this is a possibility, a urine bag should be placed in position and the infant nursed on a sheet of polyethylene.

The stools of newborn infants vary with their diet. The normal stools of breast fed infants are never formed, may be passed at hourly intervals, may contain mucus, and may be green. When lactation becomes established between the third and fifth days intestinal hurry is common, resulting in frequent stools. Later the stools tend to become less frequent and more pasty, and by the age of 3 weeks they may be passed once every two or three days. No treatment is needed. In contrast, the normal stools of bottle fed infants are formed and do not contain fluid or mucus. With certain cows' milk preparations the stools may be dark green, but this has no sinister meaning.

Acute gastroenteritis

- Dehydration
- Electrolyte abnormalities
- Cross infection

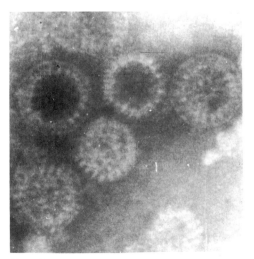

Rotavirus.

Acute gastroenteritis is an acute infection mainly affecting the small intestine that causes diarrhoea with or without vomiting. The main danger is dehydration and electrolyte imbalance, which may develop rapidly, but the infant may also be very infectious for other infants in a ward or nursery. Gastroenteritis is particularly dangerous to infants aged under 2 years.

The early signs of dehydration are often difficult to detect, but recent weight loss is often a valuable indicator. Sunken eyes, inelastic skin, and a dry tongue are late signs, but if the infant has not passed urine for several hours severe dehydration is probable. Clinical signs of dehydration are particularly difficult to detect in fat toddlers.

The infant must be examined in detail to exclude any other acute infection.

The rotavirus is the most common cause of gastroenteritis in infants and children throughout the world. It affects every age group and infection easily spreads throughout a family, although the infected adults may have few or no symptoms. Several distinct episodes of diarrhoea can be due to the rotavirus, as there are several serotypes. The incubation period is 24–48 hours and a respiratory illness, including otitis media, precedes the gastrointestinal symptoms in about half the patients. Vomiting which lasts for one to three days is followed by abnormal stools for about five days. Treatment is aimed at keeping infants well hydrated until they recover spontaneously. The frequency of the stools is reduced by dietary treatment, but the abnormal consistency of the stools persists for up to a week.

If infants are given an antibiotic early in the illness—for example, when acute otitis media is suspected as the primary diagnosis—the subsequent diarrhoea may be attributed to the antibiotic rather than to the rotavirus infection. Other drugs—for example, iron—may be associated with diarrhoea.

Management

Regrading guide for *doctors*

Total for 24 hours

Day	Volume of glucose mixture (ml)	Volume of milk (ml)	Total volume in 24 hours
1	150 × wt	0	150 × wt
2	80 × wt	70 × wt	150 × wt
3	0 × wt	150 × wt	150 × wt

No patient should receive more than 1·2 litres in 24 hours.
Feeds can be given hourly or three hourly initially and then less frequently.

Regrading guide for *mothers*

For each feed

Day	Volume of glucose mixture (ml)	Volume of milk (ml)	Total volume in each feed (ml)	No of feeds in 24 hours	Weight of infant (kg)
1	....				
2	....				
3	....				

The milk and glucose mixture should be mixed and then given to the baby.

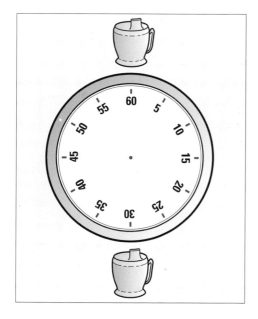

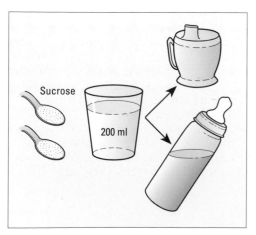

Sucrose

200 ml

Clinical signs of severe dehydration or the loss of 5% or more of body weight are definite indications for admission. If the infant relapses after treatment or there are social problems preventing treatment being carried out at home, the infant should be admitted. Infants who vomit persistently usually need to be admitted, though mild symptoms may be managed by giving frequent small volumes of liquid by mouth.

The main principle of management is to stop milk and solids, and to give a glucose or sucrose mixture. Milk is introduced after 24 hours, and this method is called regrading of feeds. Written instructions should be explained and then given to the mother. Standard forms may be helpful. Regrading may be carried out more quickly for toddlers and older children with mild symptoms. Vomiting may be reduced by giving small volumes of fluid every half hour or hour. Solids—for example, fruit or vegetable purées—should be started when the child is receiving half-strength milk.

Kaolin or Lomotil should not be prescribed, as it deflects the mother's attention from the main treatment. No antibiotics should be given to children with gastroenteritis treated at home.

Infants admitted to hospital with severe dehydration or persistent vomiting may need intravenous fluids and the withdrawal of all oral fluids for 24 hours. During the next day a third of the fluid requirement is given as oral glucose-electrolyte mixture, and later a dilute milk mixture is gradually introduced. Most infants are discharged from hospital on their normal diets within a week of admission. In hospital, infants with diarrhoea must be barrier nursed in a cubicle, which should ideally be in an annexe to the children's ward.

Rarely, a breast fed infant has gastroenteritis, but the symptoms are usually mild. The appropriate volume of rehydrating fluid is given by bottle or spoon before each breast feed.

Oral rehydrating fluids

The ideal oral rehydrating fluid is a glucose–electrolyte mixture. Single dose sachets of glucose–electrolyte powder (Dioralyte) or glucose–sucrose–electrolyte powder (Rehydrat) are available, which enable mothers to make up the mixture accurately at home. A safe alternative is 4% sucrose solution, which can be made up by the mother using 2 level teaspoonfuls of granulated sucrose in 200 ml (6 floz) water. *It is dangerous for mothers to add salt to this mixture.*

Investigations

Ideally, a stool should be sent to the laboratory for detection of pathogens, but this is not necessary for mild cases treated at home. About 15% of patients have pathogens such as campylobacter, pathogenic *Escherichia coli*, cryptosporidium, salmonella, or shigella isolated from their stools. Most cases of gastroenteritis in children are caused by viruses, usually of the rotavirus group, and these can be identified by a slide enzyme linked immunosorbent assay (ELISA) technique.

Infants needing intravenous fluids should have their plasma electrolyte and urea concentrations measured urgently.

If two or more infants in a ward or nursery have diarrhoea at the same time, even if their stool cultures show no pathogens, cross infection should be presumed. Stools from all the infants on the ward should be sent for culture and virus studies. It may be necessary to stop admissions to the ward.

- Stool culture
- ELISA rotavirus stool test
- Urine microscopy and culture
- Plasma sodium, potassium, and urea estimations

Progress and relapse

Infants must be seen again by the doctor within 12 hours of starting treatment to ensure that they are improving and not losing an excessive amount of weight, and the mother understands the management. It must be remembered that severe dehydration can occur within a few hours. It is helpful to have a specific policy to ensure adequate follow-up visits either at the family doctor's surgery or at the hospital.

The main cause of relapse or persistent symptoms is failure to follow a plan of treatment, and these patients may need to be admitted to hospital. A few infants, however, have temporary mucosal damage, which may cause intolerance to cows' milk protein or to lactose for several weeks or months (see page 45).

Causes of relapse
- Failure to follow plan
- Temporary intolerance to cows' milk protein

Gastroenteritis in developing countries

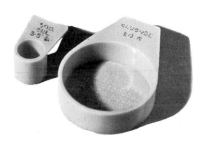

In developing countries the continuation of breast feeding during attacks of gastroenteritis may be essential for survival. Although infants who are completely breast fed rarely have severe gastroenteritis, weaning foods made up with water may infect a breast fed infant. These infants can be managed by continuing the breast feeding and supplementing the fluid intake to prevent dehydration until the infant spontaneously recovers. Supplements may be given by mouth in mild cases and intravenously in severe cases. An easier method is to give them by continuous intragastric infusion, for which the fluid does not have to be sterile.

Oral rehydrating fluids can be made up using specially designed spoons to measure the sugar and salt. Mothers and older siblings can be taught to use this mixture at the beginning of an episode of diarrhoea rather than wait until the child is dehydrated. Simple slogans such as "a cup of fluid for every stool" are effective.

INFECTION IN THE NEWBORN

Some infections are fulminating and the infant dies within a few hours. More commonly, however, the onset is insidious and the vague features may include the refusal of feeds by an infant who has fed normally, lethargy, hypotonias, apnoeic attacks, or fever. Fever is arbitrarily defined as a rectal temperature over 37·5°C, but newborn infants with infection often have a normal or even a subnormal temperature.

The most common pathogens are group B streptococci, *Escherichia coli, Staphylococcus aureus*, and *Pseudomonas*. The pathogens causing infection at a particular site can sometimes be predicted—for example, *Staph aureus* in paronychia—but swabs for bacterial culture should still be taken before giving an antibiotic. Usually an antibiotic needs to be given before the organism has been isolated, but the treatment can be changed later once the sensitivity of the pathogen to antibiotics has been tested in vitro. The sensitivity of the pathogens in a particular unit is often known, which may give a guide to effective treatment. If septicaemia is suspected and there is no obvious site of entry of the pathogen, both a penicillin and an aminoglycoside—for example, gentamicin—must be given after a blood culture has been taken.

Intestinal absorption is variable and regurgitation of antibiotics common, so that the intramuscular or intravenous route should always be used initially. Intramuscular injections should be given deeply into the upper lateral aspect of the thigh. Schemes for rotating the sites are essential to prevent local necrosis and to avoid further injections being given into a relatively avascular area. Intravenous antibiotics are given slowly by bolus injection rather than by adding them to the bottle of intravenous fluid.

Symptoms

- Refusal of feeds
- Lethargy
- Hypotonia
- Apnoea
- Fever

Group B streptococcal infections

Early onset	• Raised respiratory rate
	• Peripheral cyanosis
Late onset	• Insidious septicaemia
	• Meningitis

The group B *Streptococcus* is the commonest pathogen that causes severe infection in the first week of life. It is acquired during birth from the maternal vagina. Although about 10% of mothers are colonised and about 25% of their infants acquire this organism, only 1 in 1000 infants has symptoms. About half of those with symptoms die. In the early onset type, which occurs in the first few days of life, there may be a persistently raised respiratory rate followed by the vague features of septicaemia and later peripheral cyanosis. The chest radiograph may show extensive areas of consolidation in both lungs or it may be normal. The same organism may cause a more insidious septicaemia and meningitis towards the end of the first week.

Escherichia coli infections

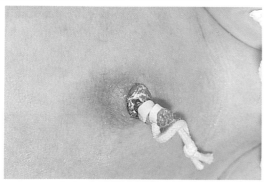
Infection of the umbilicus.

The use of antibiotics with a wide spectrum of action tends to eliminate all bacteria except *E coli* and *Pseudomonas*, which flourish in a warm, moist environment. The preterm infant, who has a greater susceptibility to infection, nursed in an incubator with increased humidity provides the ideal setting for these infections, especially if broad spectrum antibiotics are being given. The umbilicus may become infected and this may be followed by septicaemia and later meningitis.

Early symptoms are ill defined and the nurse may report that the infant appears vaguely unwell. He may have lethargy, anorexia, jaundice, and purpura. The early symptoms of meningitis are similar to those of septicaemia, but late features are vomiting, a high pitched cry, convulsions, raised anterior fontanelle tension, but rarely neck stiffness.

Infection in the newborn

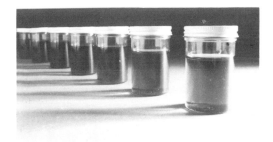

A urinary tract infection may easily be missed if a specimen of urine is not examined in every infant with fever or who is unwell. Rarely, there are physical signs of an associated congenital abnormality of the urinary tract, such as an enlarged kidney due to hydronephrosis or a persistently palpable bladder and poor urinary stream caused by obstruction from urethral valves in a boy.

Outbreaks of acute gastroenteritis due to rotavirus may occur in newborn nurseries.

Staphylococcal infections

Conjunctivitis—*Staph epidermidis* is often cultured from eye swabs of infants with conjunctivitis and it is impossible to determine whether this is the primary cause of the conjunctivitis or whether it is secondary to chemical inflammation. Chemicals, such as chlorhexidine, used in swabbing the mother's perineum may enter the infant's conjunctiva during delivery. Primary infection with *Staph aureus* may cause severe conjunctivitis. After taking an eye swab from an infant with conjunctivitis, neomycin ophthalmic ointment should be applied to both eyes three times daily for a week.

If mild conjunctivitis persists longer than a week, the possibility of infection with *Chlamydia trachomatis* should be considered. The laboratory may be able to isolate the organism using special techniques. The best treatment consists of a course of chlortetracycline eye ointment, which should be continued for at least three weeks; a course of oral erythromycin should also be given for two weeks. (See below for gonococcal conjunctivitis.)

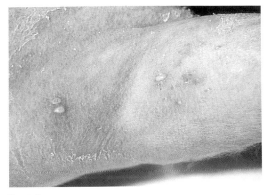

Pustules.

Skin sepsis—Clusters of yellow pustules in the axilla or groin that first appear on the fourth day or later are usually due to staphylococci. They may resemble the lesions of neonatal erythema, but those lesions appear earlier and resolve within 48 hours. If there is any doubt, the lesions should be treated as staphylococcal pustules.

Bullous impetigo of the newborn is a rare bullous eruption which can be rapidly fatal and very infectious if adequate antibiotics as intravenous flucloxacillin are not given.

Umbilical infection, shown by a localised red area and a serous exudate, may be due to *Staph aureus* or a wide variety of other pathogens.

Paronychia is an infection along the side of the nail of the fingers or toes. It often affects several digits together. The lesion appears trivial but it may lead to any of the more serious infections due to the staphylococcus. Surgery is not required but a long course of flucloxacillin should be given.

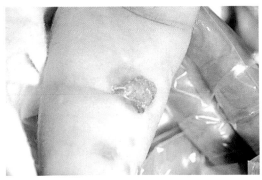

Bullous impetigo.

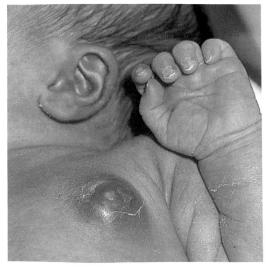

Breast abscess.

A breast abscess is a red, tender swelling, which may not affect the whole breast; usually there are enlarged lymph nodes in the axilla on the same side. Physiological enlargement may be unilateral. Surgical drainage is usually required as well as antibiotics for a breast abscess.

Pneumonia—The signs are the same as those of other types of pneumonia: raised respiratory rate, recession, and sometimes focal or generalised signs in the lungs. The infant appears extremely ill because of the accompanying septicaemia. A chest radiograph may initially show generalised non-specific changes and later lobar consolidation with characteristic pneumatocoeles, which are air filled spaces. Complications are pneumothorax and empyema.

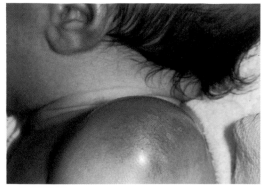

Osteomyelitis.

In *osteomyelitis* there are often no specific signs, just an ill infant who will not feed. Reluctance to move a limb and crying when the limb is moved or touched are valuable localising signs, but swelling at the site of the lesion is a late sign. A radioisotope scan may show changes at an early stage of neonatal oestomyelitis and later a radiograph of the limb may show a soft tissue swelling or a raised and thickened periosteum. Rarely osteomyelitis in the newborn is not due to *Staph aureus*.

Gonococcal infection

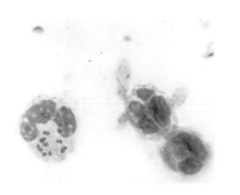

Gonococcal conjunctivitis may be unilateral, usually does not respond completely to local neomycin, and is often present within 48 hours of birth. In cases of severe conjunctivitis, particularly when bilateral and associated with severe oedema, gonococcal infection should be suspected and special arrangements for taking swabs must be made with the laboratory. If the conjunctivitis does not respond rapidly to treatment, swabs should be taken again for gonococcal infection. The paediatrician should be told as soon as the laboratory confirms the diagnosis in view of the medical and legal implications. Urethral, cervical, and rectal swabs should be taken from the mother.

If gonococcal infection is suspected, even if smears do not confirm it, intravenous penicillin is given and the diagnosis is reconsidered when the results of the cultures are available. In addition, chloramphenicol eyedrops are given half-hourly for the first six hours, and then chloramphenicol ointment is applied two-hourly for three days.

Candida infections (fungal)

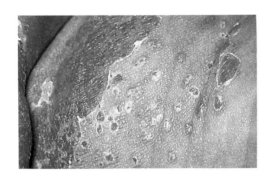

Candida infections are encouraged by the use of broad spectrum antibiotics. Candida infection of the mouth produces white plaques (thrush) and may make the infant reluctant to feed. It also causes a fiery red scaly eruption on the perineum, usually secondary to ammoniacal dermatitis. A swab made damp with sterile sodium chloride solution should be used to obtain a specimen for laboratory confirmation of the cause of the perineal rash. Oral nystatin suspension should be given after feeds for at least a week for the oral lesions. Nystatin ointment should be applied to the perineal rash each time the napkin is changed until the rash has resolved for a week. Miconazole oral gel and miconazole ointment may be used if nystatin suspension is not effective.

Management and treatment

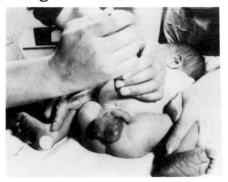

Suprapubic puncture for urine collection.

Careful evaluation of the features noted above may enable a tentative diagnosis to be made and to be confirmed by a single investigation. In many infants, however, there are no specific signs and the following investigations should be carried out.

Urine microscopy and culture—Specimens must be collected carefully and examined promptly to produce reliable results. A fresh midstream clean catch specimen can often be obtained after gentle suprapubic stimulation, especially in boys. If the urine specimen contains more than 10×10^6 pus cells per litre or bacteria are seen in a fresh specimen, a further urine specimen is obtained by suprapubic bladder puncture. Bacteria cultured from this specimen confirm a urinary tract infection.

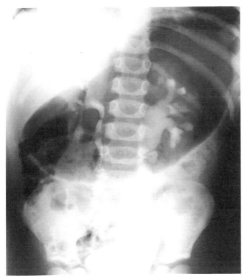

Hydronephrosis.

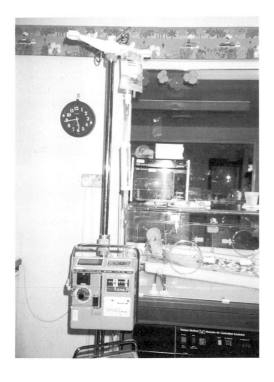

Ultrasound renal scan should be performed in all infants with a confirmed urinary tract infection before discharge from the unit. Arrangements are made for the infant to be reassessed at regular intervals in the outpatient clinic and further investigations may be needed later. Inadequately treated neonatal urinary infections may cause permanent renal scars and later renal failure.

Other investigations that may need to be performed are (*a*) culture of gastric aspirate, ear swab, and umbilical swab; (*b*) chest radiograph; (*c*) blood culture from a peripheral vein, avoiding the femoral vein; and (*d*) lumbar puncture.

After the age of 2 days a blood neutrophil polymorph count higher than $10 \times 10^9/l$ suggests infection. A very low neutrophil polymorph count also suggests overwhelming infection.

As infants may deteriorate rapidly, treatment is started immediately for the most likely organisms involved if the child is ill. If the infant appears ill, antibiotics suitable for septicaemia should be given intravenously or intramuscularly after all the specimens have been taken. If the diagnosis is uncertain after physical examination, investigation of the urine, chest radiograph, and examination of the cerebrospinal fluid (CSF), and the infant appears well, it is better to withhold antibiotics until a paediatrician has been consulted.

Suitable antibiotics are: intramuscular or intravenous flucloxacillin for staphylococcal infections; intravenous penicillin for group B streptococcal infections; and intravenous gentamicin for *E coli* septicaemia. Intravenous cefotaximine with ampicillin are suitable for *E coli* meningitis.

To treat urinary tract infection intravenous or intramuscular gentamicin and ampicillin should be given. Once the sensitivities are established it may be possible to continue treatment with one drug such as trimethoprim. In any case gentamicin should not be given for longer than a week, as eighth-nerve damage may occur. Every infant who has had a confirmed urinary tract infection should have a repeat examination of the urine for the presence of infection every three months for two years.

Gentamicin is an effective antibiotic, but it can cause deafness, and blood levels must be monitored. The serum concentrations of gentamicin should be between 5 and 10 mg/l one hour after the previous dose. The trough blood level, taken just before the next dose is due, should be less than 2 mg/l.

CONVULSIONS IN THE NEWBORN

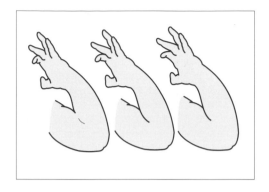

Although the involuntary movements of a convulsion are usually generalised, they may affect only one limb, the face, or tongue. The distinctive feature is repetitive jerky movements, which may be accompanied by loss of consciousness, apnoea, or rigidity. Often the convulsion has stopped by the time the baby is seen by a doctor. A brisk Moro reflex or jerky normal movements in a baby may be misinterpreted as a convulsion by an inexperienced observer. If the convulsion is not seen, apnoea or cyanosis may indicate that it has occurred, and if there is any doubt it is safer to investigate the baby on the assumption that there has been a convulsion.

Management

Exclude
(1) Hypoglycaemia
(2) Hypocalcaemia

A baby not already in hospital should be admitted. After hypoglycaemia has been excluded by a BM stix test, an anticonvulsant should be given if the convulsion is continuing or recurs while waiting for the results of other investigations. The order of carrying out the various procedures is important. Hypoglycaemia and hypocalcaemia should each be sought for and excluded in that order before the next test. Hypoglycaemia is the more dangerous condition.

The infant is placed on his side and the airway cleared by suction of the pharynx under direct vision. The baby should be nursed in an incubator to improve observation. Oxygen is given in high concentration with a funnel or head box until the convulsion has stopped.

If the plasma glucose and calcium concentrations are normal, a paediatrician should decide whether a lumbar puncture is indicated.

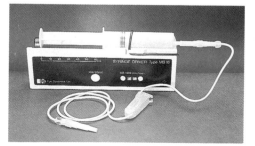

BM stix.

Hypoglycaemia

A specimen of blood should be taken from a heel prick immediately for a BM stix test. If the value is less than 2·0 mmol/l, hypoglycaemia *may* be present. A further blood sample should be taken and part of it used to repeat the BM stix test and the remainder taken into a fluoride tube for the laboratory to check the blood glucose concentration. Hypoglycaemia is defined as a laboratory estimated blood glucose level less than 2·6 mmol/l. If the second BM stix value is low, 5 ml of 10% glucose solution per kg body weight should immediately be given intravenously slowly by a scalp or limb vein. A continuous intravenous infusion of 10% glucose solution is then set up at a rate of 60 ml/kg a day.

Hypoglycaemia accompanied by fits is treated with intravenous glucose, and when the fits have ceased continuous intragastric milk should be given.

The amount of intravenous glucose should be reduced gradually over at least 24 hours. During this period three hourly BM stix tests are carried out, supplemented by regular laboratory blood glucose measurements. If an intravenous infusion of glucose is stopped suddenly by accident, severe reactive hypoglycaemia may follow and cause severe convulsions.

In contrast asymptomatic hypoglycaemia has a good prognosis. Intragastric milk should be given by continuous infusion but the milk volume should be increased by 25% to raise the blood glucose concentration. Oral or intravenous glucose should be prescribed only on the advice of a senior member of the unit. The blood glucose level is repeated an hour after starting the milk.

Milk syringe.

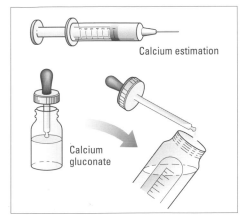

Calcium estimation

Calcium gluconate

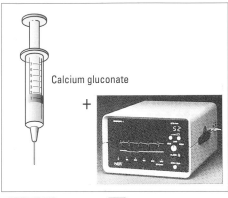

Calcium gluconate

+

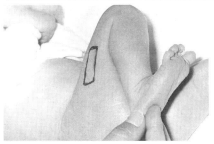

Intramuscular injection site.

Prognosis

Symptomatic hypoglycaemia: cautious prognosis

Symptomatic hypocalcaemia: good prognosis

Cerebral lesions

- Meningitis
- Cerebral oedema
- Intracranial haemorrhage

Hypocalcaemia

If the BM stix test result is normal, blood should be taken for emergency plasma calcium estimation. If convulsions are still occurring or recur after hypoglycaemia has been excluded by the BM stix test, intramuscular paraldehyde should be given while the results of detailed tests are awaited. If the plasma calcium concentration is lower than 1·8 mmol/l (7 mg/100 ml) treatment depends on whether the convulsions are still occurring or recurring. If the convulsions have stopped, 1–2 ml of 10% calcium gluconate is added to each feed. The calcium gluconate should be added to the feed and not given directly to the infant. The total dose of calcium gluconate in 24 hours should not exceed 12 ml of the 10% solution in the full-term infant.

If the convulsions continue and the plasma calcium concentration is low, 10% calcium gluconate should be diluted to 2·5% with 5% glucose solution in a syringe and given slowly intravenously into a scalp or limb vein until the convulsions cease or until a maximum of 4 ml/kg body weight of the 2·5% diluted solution has been given. The heart rate is monitored with a cardiac monitor or stethoscope during the procedure and the injection stopped if bradycardia occurs. Calcium gluconate should be added to the feeds until the plasma calcium concentration rises to normal. Calcium gluconate must never be given intramuscularly or allowed to escape out of a vein as severe tissue necrosis may occur.

Intravenous calcium may not control hypocalcaemic convulsions immediately. Some authorities have found that hypocalcaemic convulsions are treated effectively by intramuscular magnesium sulphate (0·2 ml/kg of a 10% solution/dose).

Hypomagnesaemia

In some units there is a high incidence of fits associated with low plasma magnesium concentrations. If there are recurrent fits or the plasma calcium concentration does not rise despite supplementary calcium gluconate, the plasma magnesium concentration should be estimated. If this is less than 0·6 mmol/l (1·5 mg/100 ml) intramuscular magnesium sulphate is given. The dose is 0·2 ml/kg of a 10% solution given intramuscularly every six hours; if the value is normal no further treatment is needed. The plasma estimation must be repeated after two days. The main toxic effect is hypotonia, which can be reversed by intravenous calcium gluconate if the features are severe.

Hypoglycaemia and hypocalcaemia may be found together, especially in infants of diabetic mothers, but hypoglycaemia is the more dangerous. Symptomatic hypoglycaemia may be followed by mental impairment but symptomatic hypocalcaemia or hypomagnesaemia has an excellent prognosis, although enamel hypoplasia, which predisposes to dental caries, is a late complication of hypocalcaemia. Intravenous glucose is not hazardous provided that the correct dose is given, but intravenous calcium salts may lead to cardiac arrest.

After hypoglycaemia and hypocalcaemia have been excluded, meningitis, intracranial haemorrhage, and cerebral oedema due to perinatal asphyxia should be considered. Lethargy, hypotonia, and raised tension of the anterior fontanelle are suggestive of a cerebral lesion but meningitis may be present with no specific symptoms or signs. Lumbar puncture is indicated if there is a possibility of meningitis. Ultrasound examination is reliable in excluding an intraventricular or intracerebral haemorrhage but may not detect a small subarachnoid or subdural haemorrhage.

If the first convulsion is prolonged or the convulsion recurs, intravenous phenytoin or phenobarbitone should be given. The initial dose of phenytoin or phenobarbitone is 15 mg/kg given intravenously over half an hour. The maintenance dose is started 24 hours later and is usually required for only two or three days.

WEANING

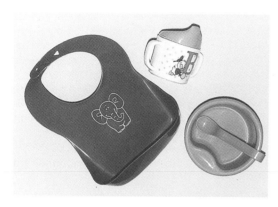

Weaning is the process of getting babies used to eating foods other than milk, and using a spoon and cup. For the first three months of life babies will need only milk and additional drinks of boiled water. New foods should start to be introduced at about 3 to 4 months. If solid foods are introduced too early babies may become too fat; if they are introduced too late, after 7 months, there may be problems with chewing. Once introduced, solid foods should be given regularly and in gradually increasing quantities. As the amount of solid food increases, the number or size of milk feeds should decrease.

Mothers need a small, wide plastic teaspoon with no sharp edges, a small plastic cup or bowl, a feeding beaker, and a cotton or plastic backed cloth bib. The feeding equipment should be kept in a sterilising solution.

Firstly, babies have to be taught to take food from the spoon rather than just sucking. As solids are increased, the volume of milk should be reduced. The baby should also be given plenty to drink to replace the milk: at least 100 to 150 ml of cooled boiled water each day. Diluted fruit juices are not necessary. Most fruit *squashes* are unsuitable for babies.

3 to 6 months

6–8 am	Milk
10 am	Milk *Baby cereal*
2 pm	Milk *Fruit or vegetable purée*
6 pm	Milk
10 pm	Milk

At 3 to 6 months babies will usually be having breast or bottle feeds at 6–8 am, 10 am, 2 pm, 6 pm, and 10 pm. Solid foods should be introduced to babies before the mid-morning or lunchtime feed—usually a baby cereal or a fruit or vegetable purée.

Mothers should start by using a cereal made from rice and should mix half to one teaspoon of cereal with one to two tablespoonfuls of breast milk, infant formula, or water; it should be given to the baby from the spoon. Sugar, honey or salt should not be added. Wheat based cereals should not be introduced until after the age of 6 months. At lunchtime babies should be fed with vegetables such as potato or carrot, or fruit such as apple. The vegetables can be fresh or frozen, and the fruit fresh or canned in natural juice. The vegetables should be boiled and the fruit stewed and then liquidised, mashed into purée or sieved. Feeding should start with half or one teaspoonful before or during the lunchtime feed and gradually increased.

At about 5 months mothers should start to give a wider variety of foods. Banana mashed with a fork is a favourite of many babies. Mashed hard boiled eggs, soups, milk puddings, and strained baby foods should all be tried, with the emphasis on savoury flavours rather than sweet ones. Lightly boiled or scrambled eggs or omelettes should *not* be given, as there is a risk of salmonella infection.

Preparing food

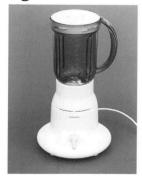

Home prepared foods are best. The mother knows what is in them and can prepare them easily and cheaply, as she can use a small portion of food cooked for the rest of the family. Many families have an electric liquidiser or food processor, but a manual blender is equally effective. A sieve is useful for making fruit and vegetable purées. If there is a deep freeze, time can be saved by preparing puréed food in bulk and storing individual portions for up to three months.

Cans, jars, and packets of baby foods are useful but should not replace home made foods. After opening, jars and cans should be kept in a refrigerator and used within 24 hours.

Iron deficiency is common during weaning but can be prevented by an appropriate diet. Iron from vegetables and cereals is not as well absorbed as that from meat. Sources of iron for vegetarians include breakfast cereals and other cereal products, pulses, green vegetables, and nut purée.

6 to 8 months

When babies are 6 months old it is no longer necessary to sterilise equipment for weaning. Bottles and teats should be sterilised until a beaker or cup is used, and that should be introduced at about this age.

At 6 to 7 months a greater variety of tastes and textures should be introduced. A little finely minced chicken, lamb, beef, or liver may be given mixed with potato purée. Vegetables should be cooked until soft, then sieved, blended or liquidised until smooth. White fish can be boiled with milk and, after the bones have been removed, mashed in with potato or vegetable purée. Dahls such as chama dahl and dhudhi, lentils and rice can be given at this age, but should not include salt or hot spices (chilli, ginger, cloves), fat or oil. Soup can be made with lentils or soft chick peas and carrots, cauliflower, or potato, which can then be blended, liquidised, or mashed. Grated cheese, cottage cheese, curd cheese, or paneer may be given, mixed in with other foods, and mashed hard boiled egg can be added to mashed potato. Babies often eat yoghurt plain, but they may need to be tempted with added fruit.

At around 7 months parents should start changing the texture of foods to encourage chewing. For example, meat and fish should be less finely minced and potatoes and other vegetables can be mashed rather than puréed. Babies should also be given hard foods such as a crust of bread, a piece of chappatti, pieces of apple, carrot, and banana, which they can hold in their hands, and this will encourage them to chew. These foods should always be given *under supervision* to make sure babies do not choke. Babies should not be given rusks or biscuits every day, as these may encourage the taste for sweet foods.

The timetable of feeds should also start to change at this age, and the number of milk feeds should fall.

Babies often reject food. This may be because they are not used to a new taste or texture. However, it may also be because they are thirsty or because the food is too hot, or simply because they want to attract attention. Mothers should be told to keep trying with new foods and to give them in different ways. Babies who become constipated should be given more fruit and vegetables and water.

At about 8 months the baby can now sit in her high chair at the table with the rest of the family. Two-course meals at lunch and teatime should be introduced—for example, a savoury food followed by a fruit purée. The amount of milk will decrease as more solids are taken. Breast feeding is continued or an infant formula milk should be given until the end of the first year.

6 am	Milk feed
9–10 am	Cereal + milk *or* hard boiled egg Milk feed
1–2 pm	Minced/puréed meat or fish, puréed vegetables and potato, gravy Diluted fruit juice or milk feed
3–4 pm	Diluted fruit juice or water
5–6 pm	Fruit purée/mashed banana Custard or milk pudding Milk feed

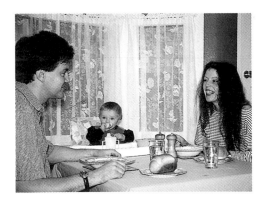

9–12 months

At this stage babies should be able to eat the same food as the rest of the family, though the food will have to be cut up or mashed. Food should not contain hot spices, particularly chilli, ginger, or cloves, and not too much butter, ghee, or oil. Each day the baby should drink a pint of milk, or less if he or she eats some cheese or yoghurt; two small portions of meat, fish, poultry, or eggs, some fruit, fresh fruit juice, or vegetables; some cereals—for example, a cereal at breakfast and half a slice of bread at tea; and a small amount of butter or margarine. Babies should not be given too many sweet foods, particularly between meals, as they can cause overweight and tooth decay.

Vitamins

Breast fed infants under 6 months do not need additional vitamins, provided the mother had an adquate vitamin status during pregnancy. From the age of 6 months infants receiving breast milk as their main drink should be given supplements of vitamins A and D.

Infants receiving 500 ml or more a day of an infant formula milk do not need vitamin supplements. Infants receiving a smaller volume of formula milk or pasteurised whole cows' milk (after the age of 1 year) should be given vitamin A and D supplements until the age of 5 years. After the age of 1 year these supplements may be omitted if the diet has an adequate vitamin content and there is moderate exposure to sunlight.

SURVEILLANCE AT 6 WEEKS

For many years, infants nursed in neonatal units have been routinely assessed at regular intervals as have those who were placed on "at risk" registers for handicaps. Total population screening was introduced when it was realised that many children later found to have disabilities were not on registers or being seen after discharge from neonatal units.

Examination of all infants at specific ages allows abnormalities to be detected at an early stage, provides mothers with a chance to discuss their anxieties, and gives opportunities for education in preventive health.

Developmental examinations should be considered on two levels: the surveillance of an apparently healthy population, and the detailed assessment of infants referred from primary examinations because of suspected abnormalities. Primary examinations, which should cover all infants in the district, are best performed by the family doctor or clinical medical officer at the community health clinic. In some districts specially trained health visitors do this work, especially for infants whose parents will not visit the surgery or clinic. Nevertheless, this system is not ideal since health visitors may consider up to 20% of infants abnormal and refer them to an assessment clinic, with all the anxiety that this entails. Some clinics are run jointly by a family doctor and health visitor, who often has wide experience of managing feeding and behaviour problems.

Infants found to be abnormal at the primary examination need to be referred to a doctor with a special interest in developmental assessment. This may be the community or the hospital paediatrician. The more detailed examination performed at this stage will probably need a team of paramedical staff.

A mother who considers that her infant has an abnormality of hearing, sight, or development must be sent straight to the specialist because she cannot be reassured until a detailed assessment has been performed, which usually needs several members of the team. The mother is likely to be right.

Primary examination

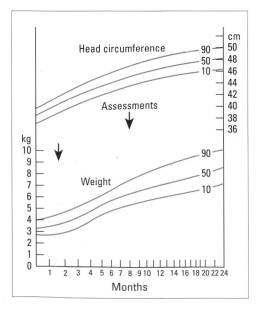

Infants in the normal population should be assessed within 48 hours of birth, at 6 weeks, and again at 7 or 8 months. Preterm infants should be examined about 6 weeks after the expected date of delivery, when their development should be the same as that of a 6 week infant born at term.

The examination should take no more than about 15 minutes and should be confined to items that have prognostic significance.

Many districts use a "parent held" manual record that, if completed correctly by professionals and parents, is a complete record of a child's health. All child health surveillance data, the dates of immunisations, and outcomes of visits to general practitioners and hospitals, and contacts with other health professionals can be recorded. Some health advice is also included throughout this record. In addition, the Health Education Authority's book *Birth to Five Years*, which is issued to all first-time mothers, is an excellent manual on child health for all parents (and junior doctors).

Review at 6 – 8 weeks

6 – 8 weeks review

For parent to complete:

This review is done by your health visitor and/or a doctor. Below is a list of things you may want to discuss when you see them. However if you are worried about your child's health, growth or development you can contact your health visitor or doctor at any time.

Health Topics for discussion:	Immunisation	☐
	Recognition of illness	☐
	Nutrition	☐
	Activities to aid development	☐
	Dangers: fire, scalds, falls, overheating	☐
Tick ☑	Good child rearing practices	☐

Circle 'Yes' or 'no' or 'not sure'

Do you feel well yourself?	Yes/no/not sure
Do you have any worries about **feeding** your baby?	Yes/no/not sure
Do you have any concerns about your baby's **weight** gain?	Yes/no/not sure
Does your baby watch your face and follow with his/her eyes?	Yes/no/not sure
Does your baby turn towards the light?	Yes/no/not sure
Does your baby smile at you?	Yes/no/not sure
Do you think your baby can hear you?	Yes/no/not sure
Is your baby startled by loud noises?	Yes/no/not sure
Are there any problems in looking after your baby?	Yes/no/not sure
Do you have any other worries about your baby?	Yes/no/not sure
Comment _____	

How are you feeding your baby?   Breast/Bottle/mixed

Keep hot drinks away from children. Use a coiled-flex kettle.

Check the water before you bath your baby. Hot water can scald your baby badly.

Review at 6 – 8 weeks

* Please place a sticker (if available) otherwise write in space provided.

Surname ☐☐☐☐☐☐☐☐☐☐☐☐☐☐
First names ☐☐☐☐☐☐☐☐☐☐☐☐☐☐
NHS number ☐☐☐☐☐☐ Local no ☐☐☐☐☐☐
Address _____ Sex M/F
_____ Postcode _____ D.O.B. __/__/__
G.P. ☐☐☐☐☐☐☐☐ Code ☐☐☐☐☐☐
H.V. ☐☐☐☐☐☐☐☐ Code ☐☐☐☐☐☐

Date of Examination _____ / _____ / _____
Age in weeks _____
Name of Examiner ☐☐☐☐☐☐☐☐☐☐☐☐☐☐☐☐
Examiner Code number ☐☐☐☐☐☐   Examination centre ☐☐☐☐☐
WEIGHT _____ kg _____ centile
HEAD CIRC. _____ cm _____ centile
FEEDING _____ Breast/Bottle/Mixed

Any previous ongoing medical problems?   No ☐   Yes ☐
If 'yes' please specify   (1) _____   (2) _____   (3) _____
ICD Code ☐☐☐☐☐☐☐   ☐☐☐☐☐☐☐   ☐☐☐☐☐☐☐

ITEM	GUIDE TO CONTENT	CODE (Ring one)*	COMMENT
Physical	Full physical exam. Fontanelles. Palate. Skin	S P O T R N	
Vision	Eyes. Follows. Red reflex.	S P O T R N	
Hearing	Ears. Risk factor. Parents observations	S P O T R N	
Locomotion	Tone, movement, reflexes	S P O T R N	
Manipulation	Moro and grasp	S P O T R N	
Speech/Lang.	Vocalisation	S P O T R N	
Behaviour	Social smile. Cry. Sleep	S P O T R N	
Hips	and skeletal system	S P O T R N	
Genitalia		S P O T R N	
Heart	Femoral pulses	S P O T R N	

*(If one or more codes seem to apply select the last one e.g. R takes priority over T, T over O etc.)

S = Satisfactory *(normal result)*
P = Problem *(significant condition on record)*
O = Observation *(special recall arranged)*
T = Treatment or investigation underway
R = Referred to any community or hospital service
N = Not examined for this item

Referred to (1) _____ (2) _____
(3) _____
Special recall in _____ wks/mths   Signature _____

White copy: Stay in Record   Yellow copy: to Child Health Office
Pink copy: to GP/HV

6 – 8 weeks

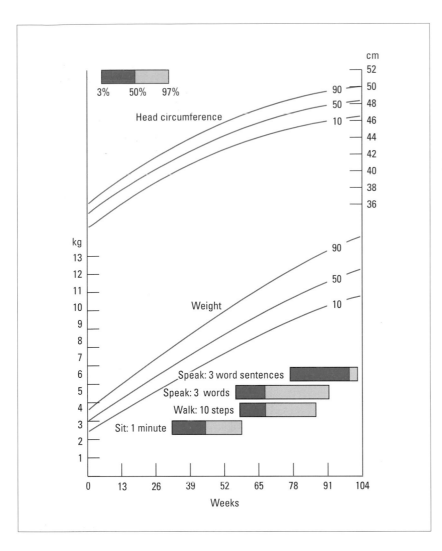

3% | 50% | 97%

Head circumference

cm
52
50
48
46
44
42
40
38
36

90
50
10

kg
13
12
11
10
9
8
7
6
5
4
3
2
1

90
50
10

Weight

Speak: 3 word sentences

Speak: 3 words

Walk: 10 steps

Sit: 1 minute

0   13   26   39   52   65   78   91   104

Weeks

The 6 week examination should include a physical examination and assessment of alertness, vision, and motor function. The checks should be carried out as part of clinical care and not be regarded as pass or fail examinations. A simple form is useful for recording the information quickly. Screening for hearing defects is not usually done until 7 or 8 months, and other abilities are assessed more sporadically, depending on whether the mother takes the child to a local clinic or to the general practitioner's special baby clinic.

Of greatest importance is the child's alertness, interest in his surroundings, responsiveness, and ability to concentrate.

The physical examination of the infant should always include measurement of weight and head circumference. These values, plotted on a growth chart, will show at a glance whether the infant's growth is normal.

Vision and squint

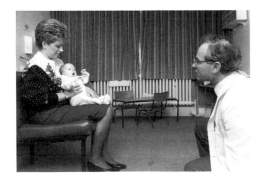

The infant's visual attention is engaged by the examiner crouching about 60 cm in front of the infant so that their eyes are on the same level. When the examiner slowly moves his head a short distance to one side then the other, the normal infant will continue to hold his gaze. Failure to do so is abnormal but may be due to something distracting the infant. Infants who fail to follow must be examined again two weeks later. Possible causes include lack of stimulation at home, delay in development, or blindness.

The second routine test at this age is the detection of the red reflex. If a bright ophthalmoscope is held about 45 cm away from an infant's eye, with the observer looking down the beam of light, a bright red reflex is normally seen in a fair skinned infant, and a dark red or grey reflex in an infant with a dark skin. Absence of the reflex indicates an abnormality of the refractive media and requires urgent referral to an opthalmologist.

An infant who does not fixate on the examiner's face at the second visit should be referred to a developmental specialist. At that stage additional tests will include an attempt to determine whether the infant can see at all by showing him a revolving Catford drum. This induces opticokinetic nystagmus—an involuntary movement of the eyes, which occurs even if the infant does not concentrate well.

In a young infant a squint can be noticed by observing the position of the light reflex on each cornea when a torch is shone into the eyes. Normally the reflex should be in the centre of each pupil or at a corresponding point on each cornea. If there is a possibility of a squint, movements of the eyes should be assessed and the cornea, lens, and fundi should be examined. An infant with a squint needs to be referred to an ophthalmologist.

Motor function

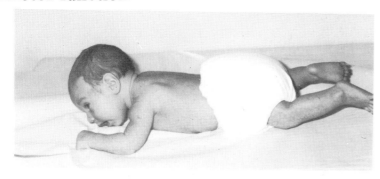

The baby should be placed prone on a couch; normally he will lift his head for a few seconds, though some infants may take a few minutes to do so. Infants who usually sleep prone are more advanced in lifting their heads than others. If the infant does not eventually lift his head he needs to be re-examined two weeks later.

When the infant is held in the prone position, his head rises to the same plane as his trunk and his legs do *not* fall vertically.

Other assessments

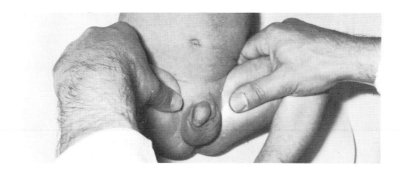

The testes and hips should be examined by the methods described for the newborn infant. It is difficult to detect an abnormal hip at the age of 6 weeks and ideally the condition should have been detected in the newborn infant.

Cardiac murmurs should be sought for and the femoral pulses checked. Though hearing is not tested at 6 weeks, the normal infant will respond to sounds by stopping crying, opening his eyes widely or by a startle reflex, depending on the intensity of the sound.

Patterns of development in childhood

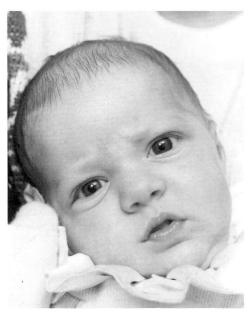

Looking at the camera.

Progress in a particular field does not occur gradually but in spurts, and when one skill is advancing quickly others tend to go into abeyance.

There is considerable variation in the range of normal development, but among the children who fall outside the normal range there are some who later turn out to be normal. The children who fall into this group need examining more closely and more often to determine which are definitely abnormal. They should be referred to developmental specialists.

Lack of appropriate stimulation may cause delay in physical, intellectual, or social development. This factor must be taken into account if the child has been cared for in an institution or if the mother has a learning disability or has had puerperal depression. These children advance rapidly when the mother is given advice on handling them or they are placed in a better environment. Delayed speech development, probably the commonest disability of childhood, may be prevented by encouraging mothers to talk to their infants from birth.

No child has impaired intelligence if development is delayed in a single field and normal in all others. A child who is slow at learning will be delayed in all fields, except sometimes in walking. Intelligence cannot be assessed accurately until the age of about $4\frac{1}{2}$ years and before that age it is best to use the term developmental delay.

SURVEILLANCE AT 8 MONTHS

Mothers are asked whether they have any problems and whether the infants have had any illnesses since the last examination. They are also asked whether the infants are making sounds and the details of their diet, in particular whether they are chewing solids.

As at 6 weeks, the infant's alertness and interest are checked. Head circumference and weight should be measured and plotted on the growth chart.

Vision

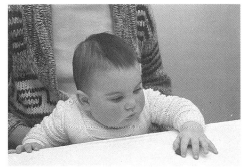

Near vision being tested.

Eye movements should be noted. If a squint is suspected, the position of the light reflex in each cornea should be observed; if there is a squint, the reflex will be in a different position in each eye. While the infant looks at an object one eye is covered with the doctor's hand. If the eye that is not being covered moves to fixate the object, that eye has an overt squint. The covering hand is slowly removed and if that eye moves to fixate the object, there is a latent squint. If a squint is seen or suspected at any time the infant should be seen by an ophthalmologist.

Near vision may be tested by placing a raisin or pellet of paper about 20 cm in front of an infant and watching whether he reaches out to grab it. Testing distant vision is time-consuming at this age and is usually performed only at specialist clinics.

Motor development

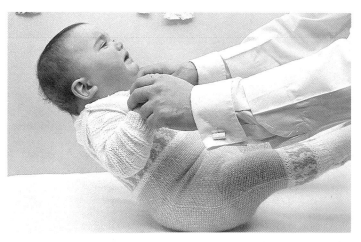

From the prone position infants should get up on their wrists. When pulled from the supine position they should be able to sit spontaneously for a minute or two. Normal children can sit without help by the age of 8 months. Infants should also be able to take their weight on their legs when they are held standing.

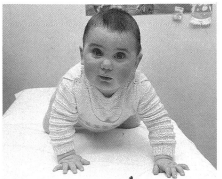

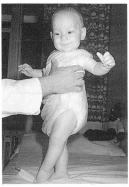

Review at 8 – 9 months
For parent to complete

Health Topics for discussion: Tick ☑	Accident prevention: choking, scalds, safety in cars and house, sunburn **Dental advice** **Developmental needs** **Nutrition, etc**

This review is done by your health visitor and/or a doctor. Below is a list of things you may want to discuss when you see them. However if you are worried about your child's health, growth or development you can contact your health visitor or doctor at any time.

Circle 'Yes' or 'no' or 'not sure'

Are you feeling well yourself?	Yes/no/not sure
Have you any worries about your child's health?	Yes/no/not sure
Do you have any worries about how your baby is feeding?	Yes/no/not sure
Are you happy your baby is gaining weight?	Yes/no/not sure
Do you have any worries about your baby's development? (see pages 12 – 13)	Yes/no/not sure
Is your baby sitting alone?	Yes/no/not sure
Is your baby using both hands?	Yes/no/not sure
Does your baby babble (Ba-ba, da-da etc)?	Yes/no/not sure
Have you any worries about your baby's eyesight?	Yes/no/not sure
Can s/he recognise carer at a distance?	Yes/no/not sure
Have you noticed a squint (eyes not moving together?)	Yes/no/not sure
Do you think your baby can hear you?	Yes/no/not sure
Comment _____
_____

Are all your child's immunisations up to date   Yes/no

Do you have fire guards to stop your child touching heaters and open fires?

Review at 8 – 9 months
* Please place a sticker (if available) otherwise write in space provided.

Surname [ ]
First names [ ]
NHS number [ ]   Local no [ ]
Address _____   Sex M/F
_____ Postcode _____ D.O.B. __/__/__
G.P. [ ] Code [ ]
H.V. [ ] Code [ ]

Date of Examination _____ / _____ / _____
Age in months _____
Name of Examiner [ ]
Examiner Code number [ ]   Examination centre [ ]
WEIGHT _____ kg _____ centile
HEAD CIRC. _____ cm _____ centile

Any previous ongoing medical problems?   No ☐   Yes ☐
If 'yes' please specify   (1) _____   (2) _____   (3) _____
ICD Code [ ]   [ ]   [ ]

ITEM	GUIDE TO CONTENT	CODE (Ring one)*	COMMENT
Physical	Parents observations. Diet.	S P O T R N	
Vision	Eye movements. Visual behaviour. Cover test.	S P O T R N	
Hearing	Distraction Test.	S P O T R N	
Locomotion	Sitting. Some weight bearing.	S P O T R N	
Manipulation	Transfers. Uses both hands.	S P O T R N	
Speech/Lang.	Babble. Responds to speech.	S P O T R N	
Behaviour	Knows strangers. Enjoys mirror image. Socialisation Alertness.	S P O T R N	
Hips	Check for CDH	S P O T R N	
Genitalia	Testicular descent (Ring 'N' for girl)	S P O T R N	
Heart		S P O T R N	

*(If one or more codes seem to apply select the last one e.g. R takes priority over T, T over O etc.)

S = Satisfactory *(normal result)*
P = Problem *(significant condition on record)*
O = Observation *(special recall arranged)*
T = Treatment or investigation underway
R = Referred to any community or hospital service
N = Not examined for this item

Referred to (1)_____ (2) _____
(3) _____
Special recall in _____ wks/mths   Signature _____

White copy: Stay in Record   Yellow copy: to Child Health Office
Pink copy: to GP/HV

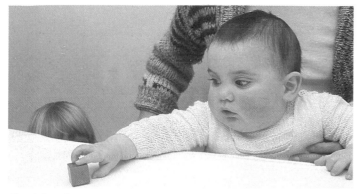

Hand function.

If a cube is placed in front of the infant he should grab it with his whole hand. This test should be tried for both the right and the left hand, and the infant should transfer the object from one hand to the other. Infants who perform all these tests normally but are not sitting spontaneously should be seen again two months later.

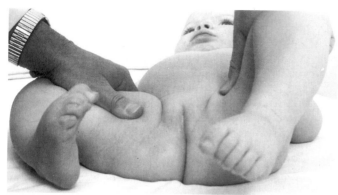

Testing hips.

A dislocated hip will show reduction of abduction and a proximal displacement of the lower buttock crease. Bilateral dislocation is hard to detect clinically but radiographs of the hips will confirm the diagnosis at this age.

Hearing

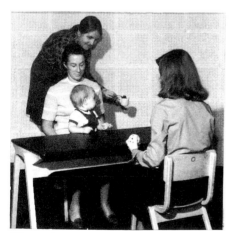

Distraction test.

The distraction method is the hearing test used at this age. The distractor holds the infant's attention while the tester produces a sound. Careful attention to detail is essential to produce reliable results. The mother is requested to position the infant at the edge of her lap and not to react to the sounds. The distractor sits at the level of the infant's face and holds the infant's attention with a toy that produces no noise. Eye contact is avoided. The toy is withdrawn from sight and immediately afterwards the tester produces the test sound at a distance of 45 cm from the infant's ear, on a level with the ear, but slightly behind it so that the infant does not see the test object or the tester's shadow. The distractor detects whether the infant turns the head or eyes abruptly towards the sound. The speed with which the infant responds to the sound is a useful indication of his alertness. The test sounds should include those with a known pitch and intensity such as a warbler. Voice sounds at minimal intensity should include "psss," "phth" (for high tones), or "oo" (for low tones). If an infant fails to turn to the sound, the ability to turn the head to each side should be assessed. If the infant responds to sounds on two out of three tests performed on one ear, hearing is considered normal in that ear. If the infant fails to respond, the ears should be examined with an auriscope.

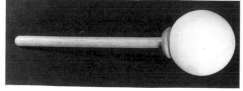

High-pitched rattle.

The room where the test is performed must be quiet. It should ideally have a carpet and be removed from the waiting area and sounds of traffic. The commonest reasons for a child failing to respond to the test sounds are lack of interest, tiredness, distraction, wax blocking the external meatus, otitis media, and lack of familiarity with the test sounds. It is important to explain to the mother that these are far more likely reasons for lack of response than deafness, and that the test will be repeated by the same person one month later. Infants who fail to respond at the second visit should be seen by an audiologist.

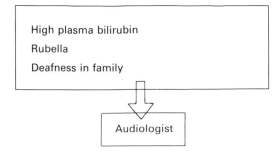

High plasma bilirubin

Rubella

Deafness in family

→ Audiologist

High tone deafness cannot be excluded by these tests and if there is a high suspicion of deafness—for example, if the infant had a very high plasma bilirubin concentration in the neonatal period, has rubella syndrome, or has a family history of deafness—the infant should be seen by an audiologist even if the results of these simple tests appear normal. Pure tone audiology may be needed, and the audiologist may have to see the child several times before a hearing defect can be completely excluded.

Pattern of development

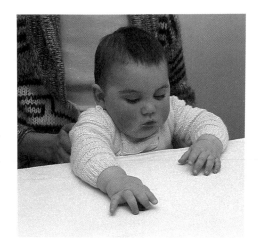

Most normal children sit unaided by the age of 8 months. African children tend to advance in most aspects of development faster than other children up to the age of about 7 months. In some families one aspect of development—for example, sitting, walking, or speech—may be unusually early or late, the development in all other fields being normal.

Finding that an infant is not sitting by a certain age does not necessarily mean that he is abnormal, as he may have a variation of normal development. These children fall into a group who are late in reaching a developmental milestone, and it is reasonable that they should be referred for further examination to exclude more sinister problems.

RESPIRATORY INFECTIONS IN THE OLDER INFANT

Infection of the respiratory tract is a common cause of illness of infants. Although pathogens are often not confined to anatomical boundaries, the infections may be classified as: (*a*) upper respiratory tract —common cold, tonsillitis, and otitis media; (*b*) middle respiratory tract—acute laryngitis and epiglottitis; (*c*) lower respiratory tract—bronchitis, bronchiolitis, and pneumonia.

Upper respiratory tract infection is usually the least serious condition but blockage of the nose by mucus may completely obstruct the airway in those infants who cannot breathe through their mouths. Middle respiratory tract infection may totally obstruct airflow at the narrowest part of the airway. Lower respiratory tract infection produces trivial signs initially but may be lethal within a few hours.

Viruses, which cause most respiratory tract infections, and bacterial infections produce similar clinical illness. Different viruses may produce an identical clinical picture, or the same virus may cause different clinical syndromes. Clinically it may not be possible to determine whether the infection is due to viruses, bacteria, or both. If the infection is suspected of being bacterial, it is safest to prescribe an antibiotic, as the results of virus studies are often received after the acute symptoms have passed. The commonest bacterial pathogens are pneumococci, *Haemophilus influenzae*, group A β haemolytic streptococci, and *Staphylococcus aureus*. Group B streptococci, Gram negative bacteria, and anaerobic bacteria are less common.

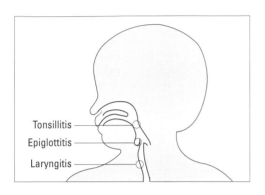

Common cold (coryza)

Preschool children have at least three to six colds each year. The main symptoms are sneezing, nasal discharge, cough, and, rarely, fever. Nasal obstruction in infants who cannot breathe through their mouths may cause feeding difficulties and, rarely, brief periods of apnoea. Similar symptoms may occur in the early phases of infection with rotavirus and be followed by vomiting and diarrhoea. Postnasal discharge may produce coughing. The commonest complication is acute otitis media, but secondary bacterial infection of the lower respiratory tract sometimes occurs.

There is no specific treatment for the common cold, and antibiotics should be avoided. If an infant is not able to feed due to nasal obstruction from mucus, two drops of 0·9% sodium chloride solution can be instilled into each nostril before feeds three times daily. This will wash the mucus into the back of the pharynx and relieve the obstruction. There is a danger with nasal drops that they will run down into the lower respiratory tract and carry the infection there.

Main symptoms
- Sneezing
- Nasal discharge
- Cough
- Fever (rare)

Tonsillitis and pharyngitis

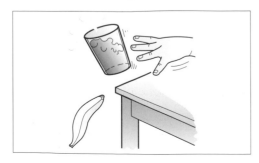

In children aged under 3 years the commonest presenting features of tonsillitis are fever and refusal to eat, but a febrile convulsion may occur at the onset. Older children may complain of a sore throat or enlarged cervical lymph nodes, which may or may not be painful. Viral and bacterial causes cannot be distinguished clinically as a purulent follicular exudate may be present in both. Ideally, a throat swab should be sent to the laboratory before starting treatment, to determine a bacterial cause for the symptoms and to help to indicate the pathogens currently in the community. There has been a recurrence of group A haemolytic streptococci in outbreaks of sore throat and a more liberal

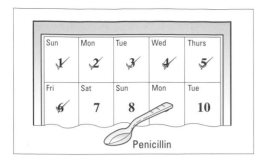

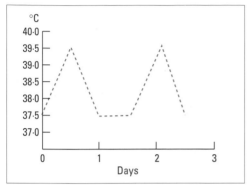

use of penicillin is justified. As this organism is the only important bacterium causing tonsillitis, penicillin is the drug of choice and the only justification for using another antibiotic is a convincing history of hypersensitivity to penicillin. In that case the alternative is erythromycin. In the absence of an outbreak of group A streptococcus infection the indication for oral penicillin is fever or severe systemic symptoms. The drug should be continued for at least 10 days if a streptococcal infection is confirmed. Parents often stop the drug after a few days as the symptoms have often abated and the medicine is unpalatable. The organism is not eradicated unless a full 10-day course is given.

Viral infections often produce two peaks on the temperature chart.

An extensive thick white shaggy exudate on the tonsils (sometimes invading the pharynx) suggests infectious mononucleosis, and a full blood count, examination of the blood film, and a Monospot test are indicated. A membranous exudate on the tonsils suggests diphtheria and an urgent expert opinion should be sought.

Fluids can be given while there is dysphagia, and regular paracetamol during the first 24 to 48 hours reduces fever and discomfort.

A peritonsillar abscess (quinsy) is now extremely rare. It displaces the tonsil medially so that the swollen soft palate obscures the tonsil and the uvula is displaced across the midline. The advice of an otolaryngology surgeon is needed urgently.

Otitis media

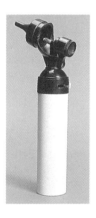

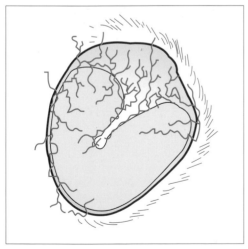

Pain is the main symptom of acute otitis media and is one of the few causes of a fretful infant who cries all night. The pain is relieved if the media drum ruptures. Viruses probably cause over half the cases of acute otitis, but a vital or bacterial origin cannot be distinguished clinically. The commonest bacteria are pneumococci, group A β haemolytic streptococci, and *H influenzae*.

Children are often fascinated by the light of the auriscope, and the auriscope speculum can be placed on a doll or the child's forearm for reassurance. Gentleness is essential and the speculum should never be pushed too far into the external meatus because this cases pain. If the pinna is pulled gently outwards and downwards to open the meatal canal, the tympanic membrane is visible with the tip of the speculum in the outer end of the meatus. In early cases of otitis media there are dilated vessels over the upper and posterior part of the drum. Later, the tympanic membrane becomes red, congested, and bulging and the light reflex is lost. Swelling or tenderness behind the pinna should always be sought, as mastoiditis can be easily missed.

The choice of initial treatment lies between amoxycillin and erythromycin. If there is no improvement in the drums after two or three days, another antibiotic should be substituted. Cefaclor or amoxycillin with clavulanic acid may be included in the second line drugs. The duration of the course of antibiotics is controversial. The most common view is that antibiotics should be given for at least 10 days and the ears examined again before the course is stopped. There is some evidence that short courses of 3–5 days of antibiotics given at high doses may be as effective as the longer courses. Ideally, a hearing test should be performed a few months after each attack of acute otitis media to detect residual deafness and "glue ear". One study showed that after the first attack of acute otitis media in infants, which was treated with antimicrobial agents, 40% of patients had no middle ear effusion after one month and 90% after three months.

Stridor

Stridor is noisy breathing caused by obstruction in the pharynx, larynx, or trachea. It may be distinguished from partial obstruction of the bronchi by the absence of rhonchi. Although most cases are due to acute laryngitis and may resolve with the minimum of care, similar features may be due to a foreign body and may cause sudden death.

Stridor is recognised as one of the most ominous signs in childhood. Any doctor should be able to recognise the sound over the telephone and arrange to see the child immediately. Examination of the throat may precipitate total obstruction of the airway and should be attempted only in the presence of an anaesthetist and facilities for intubation.

A glance at the child will show whether urgent treatment is needed or whether there is time for a detailed history to be taken. The doctor needs to know when the symptoms started and whether there is nasal discharge or cough. Choking over food, especially peanuts, or the abrupt onset of symptoms after playing alone with small objects suggests that a foreign body is present.

During the taking of the history and the examination mothers should remain near their children and be encouraged to hold them and to talk to them. All unpleasant procedures, such as venepuncture, should be avoided. This reduces the possibility of struggling, which may precipitate complete airway obstruction. Agitation and struggling raise the peak flow rate and move secretions, which results in increased hypoxia and the production of more secretions.

```
Throat examination
                       ↘
Venepuncture           →  Cardiac arrest
                       ↗
Struggling
```

Acute laryngotracheitis

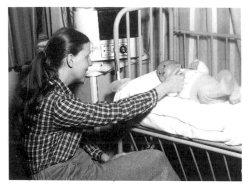

Humidifier in background.

Acute laryngitis causes partial obstruction of the larynx. It is characterised by inspiratory and expiratory stridor (noisy breathing), cough, and hoarseness. The laryngeal obstruction is due to oedema, spasm, and secretions. Affected children are usually aged 6 months to 3 years, and the symptoms are most severe in the early hours of the morning. Recession of the intercostal spaces indicates significant obstruction, and cyanosis or drowsiness shows that total obstruction of the airway is imminent.

Restless

- Hypoxia
- Thirst
- Hunger
- Fear

A child often improves considerably after inhaling steam, which is provided easily by turning on the hot taps in the bathroom. Mild cases may be treated successfully at home using this method, but children must be visited every few hours to determine whether they are deteriorating and need to be admitted to hospital. Continuous stridor or recession demands urgent hospital admission. Hypoxaemia or thirst may cause restlessness and should be corrected and sedatives avoided. Rarely, the obstruction needs to be relieved by passing an endotracheal tube or performing a tracheostomy.

Acute laryngotracheitis is usually caused by a viral infection and therefore infants with mild symptoms do not need antibiotics. In a few cases *Staph aureus* or *H influenzae* is present and the associated septicaemia makes the child appear very ill. Bacterial infection is characterised by plaques of debris and pus on the surface of the trachea, partially obstructing it, just below the vocal cords. Acute epiglottitis and acute laryngitis may be indistinguishable clinically since stridor and progressive upper airway obstruction are the main features of both. If bacterial infection is suspected cefotaxime is given intravenously. Some paediatricians give steroids as well. The dose of hydrocortisone is 100 mg intramuscularly or intravenously repeated once after two hours. No effect is seen for at least two hours. Later, betamethasone should be given at a dose of 3 mg intravenously every six hours but only until signs of improvement appear. Children with severe symptoms should be managed in the intensive care unit.

Children with epiglottitis are usually aged over 2 years; drooling and dysphagia are common, and the child usually wants to sit upright. When the obstruction is very severe, the stridor becomes ominously quieter. There is usually an associated septicaemia with *H influenzae*.

Transcutaneous blood oxygen saturation monitor.

Other causes of stridor

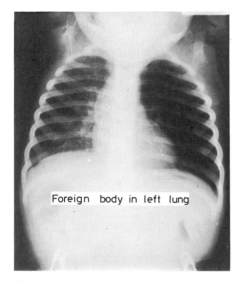

Hypertranslucent left lung due to foreign body.

Even if the symptoms have settled and there are no abnormal signs, a history of the onset of sudden choking or coughing can never be ignored. A radiograph of the neck and chest should be taken and may show a hypertranslucent lung obstructed by a foreign body, a shift of the mediastinum, or, less commonly, collapse of part of the lung or a radio-opaque foreign body. The radiograph may be considered normal. Bronchoscopy may be needed to exclude a foreign body even if the chest radiograph appears to be normal. Stridor in a child who has had scalds or burns or has inhaled steam from a kettle suggests that intubation or tracheostomy may be needed urgently.

If the cause of stridor is likely to be a foreign body below the larynx, the object should be removed immediately by a thoracic surgeon in the main or accident and emergency operating theatre. If the object is above the larynx and if an ENT surgeon or anaesthetist is not immediately available and the child is deteriorating, the safest treatment is to insert a wide needle, such as Medicut size 14, into the trachea in the midline just below the thyroid cartilage. It may be preferable to insert two needles. No attempt should be made to look at the mouth or throat or remove the object, as the struggling that may follow may impact the object and prove fatal. A first aid measure usually performed before arrival is to slap the infant's back between the shoulder blades while holding the infant upside down by the legs. The child should remain in the position he or she finds most comfortable, which is usually upright. Forceful attempts to make the child lie flat—for example, for a radiograph—may result in complete airway obstruction.

Infants with congenital laryngeal stridor, which is due to loose aryepiglottic folds, usually have inspiratory stridor only. The symptoms begin during the first few weeks of life and usually persist for several months, becoming more severe during episodes of upper respiratory tract infections or while crying, but subsiding in sleep.

Acute bronchitis

Upper limit for normal respiratory rate related to age	
<2 months	60/min
2–11 months	50/min
12–60 months	40/min

Acute bronchitis often follows a viral upper respiratory tract infection; there is always a cough, which may be accompanied by wheezing. There is no fever or difficulty with feeding. The respiratory rate is normal and the symptoms resolve within a week. The only signs, which are not always present continuously, are rhonchi. Since bronchitis is usually due to a virus, antibiotics are indicated only if secondary bacterial infection is suspected.

Acute bronchiolitis

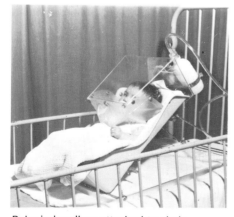

Baby in headbox attached to chair.

Acute bronchiolitis is an acute infection that occurs in winter epidemics in infants aged under 1 year. For the first few days there may be only a rasping cough but deterioration may occur within a few hours, causing a raised respiratory rate, indrawing of the intecostal spaces, cyanosis, drowsiness, and apparent enlargement of the liver. The respiratory syncytial virus is found in over 70% of cases. During epidemics the disease may be recognised at an early stage, but at the beginning of epidemics the condition may be recognised only when the infant is moribund. Signs in the chest vary at different stages of the illness and there may be no adventitious sounds. The chest radiograph may appear normal even in severely ill infants. In units with ELISA or immunofluorescence techniques for diagnosing respiratory syncytial virus, results are available the same day, treatment can be planned, and cross infection avoided. Oxygen is the most important aspect of treatment and is efficiently given by a headbox attached to a chair. Most infants need intragastric tube feeding or intravenous fluids for a few days. Where a viral cause can be confirmed immediately, antibiotics can be avoided. But they should not be withheld from severely ill infants, as there is a possibility of additional bacterial infection. A few infants develop progressive respiratory distress, and intermittent positive pressure ventilation may have to be considered. The value of ribavirin, an antiviral agent, is being assessed.

The infant is discharged from hospital when feeding is normal. The cough may persist for six weeks, but if there is no improvement after three weeks, a sweat test should be performed to exclude cystic fibrosis.

Bronchopneumonia and segmental pneumonia

Pneumonia is acute inflammation of the lung alveoli. In bronchopneumonia the infection is spread throughout the bronchial tree whereas in segmental pneumonia it is confined to the alveoli in one segment or lobe. A raised respiratory rate at rest or indrawing of the intercostal spaces distinguishes pneumonia from bronchitis. The upper limit for a normal respiratory rate is related to age (see page 77). Cough, fever, and flaring of the alae nasi are usually present and there may be reduced breath sounds over the affected area as well as crepitations. A chest radiograph, which is needed for every child with suspected pneumonia, may show extensive changes when there are no localising signs in the chest. The radiograph may show an opacity confined to a single segment or lobe, but there may be bilateral patchy changes. Bacterial cultures of throat swabs and blood should be performed before treatment is started. Ideally, nasopharyngeal secretions should be studied virologically and virus antibody titres of serum collected in the acute and convalescent phases should be measured.

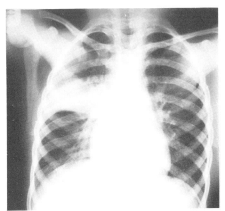

Chest radiograph showing pneumonia in the right lung.

Children with pneumonia are best treated in hospital, as they may need oxygen treatment. Antibiotics should be prescribed for all cases of pneumonia, although a viral cause may be discovered later. If the child is not vomiting and not severely ill, oral erythromycin or amoxycillin is given. Cefotaxime is given intravenously if the symptoms are severe, and erythromycin is added when failure to improve promptly suggests infection with mycoplasma or chlamydia. Antibiotic treatment can be modified when the results of bacterial cultures are available. Intravenous fluids may be needed.

The chest radiograph of a child with segmental or lobar pneumonia should be repeated after one month.

Recurrent respiratory infections

Although all doctors concerned with children are familiar with the catarrhal child, the exact pathology of the condition is unknown, and it is called by many names—postnasal discharge, perennial rhinitis, or recurrent bronchitis. These children have an increased incidence of colds, tonsillitis, and acute otitis media. Recurrent episodes of symptoms such as fever, nasal discharge, and cough are most common during the second half of the first year of life, the first two years at nursery school, and the first two years at primary school. Recurrent viral or bacterial infections contracted from siblings or fellow pupils may be important, but the considerable differences between the behaviour of children in the same family suggest the possibility of a temporary immunological defect.

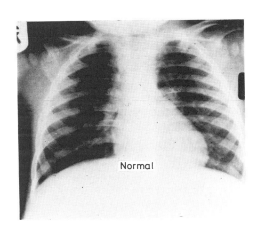

Normal

Various treatments including nasal drops and oral preparations of antihistamines are given with little effect. A chest radiograph should be performed to exclude persistent segmental or lobar collapse. A sweat test should be carried out to exclude cystic fibrosis, and plasma immunoglobulin studies should be conducted to exclude rare syndromes.

Recurrent bronchitis

Recurrent Bronchitis
?
Bronchial asthma

Two separate episodes of acute bronchitis may occur in a normal child in a year. If attacks are more frequent at any age, bronchial asthma should be considered. Viruses cause the majority of attacks of bronchitis and will precipitate most attacks of bronchial asthma. Some paediatricians have reverted recently to the older terms recurrent or wheezy bronchitis, as most children with these features become free of symptoms by the age of 5. Although the pathological processes and prognosis may differ between recurrent bronchitis and bronchial asthma, there is no clinical or laboratory method of distinguishing between them and treatment is the same.

After an episode of severe symptoms during an infection with respiratory syncytial virus (bronchiolitis), many children have recurrent

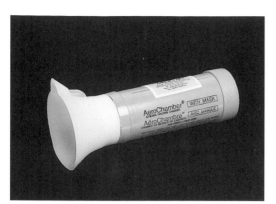

episodes of cough and wheezing during the subsequent four years. It is not known whether the respiratory syncytial virus predisposes the child to recurrent respiratory symptoms or whether the child has a predisposition to produce severe symptoms with viral respiratory infections.

If there is a persistent or recurrent cough, a chest radiograph should be performed to exclude persistent segmental or lobar collapse. A Mantoux test for tuberculosis and a sweat test to exclude cystic fibrosis should be performed, and plasma concentrations of immunoglobulins and IgG subclasses should be measured to exclude transient or permanent immune deficiencies.

The management of recurrent bronchitis or bronchial asthma is the same. For infants with mild symptoms an oral bronchodilator, for example salbutamol, can be given at the beginning of an episode and continued for a week. If this is not effective, a bronchodilator can be given by air pump and nebuliser or a *small* spacer device with a face mask. Infants with severe or frequent episodes can be given a prophylactic drug starting with sodium cromoglycate and changing to an inhaled steroid if there is no improvement after six weeks. Prophylactic drugs can be given by an air pump and nebuliser or with a small spacer device. If infants are receiving both a bronchodilator and a prophylactic drug, the dose of bronchodilator should be given just before the prophylactic drug.

FEVER IN THE OLDER INFANT

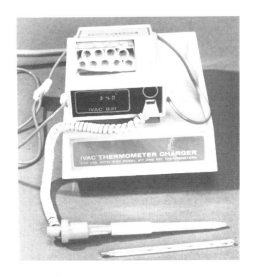

The normal oral or rectal temperature is about 37·5°C (99·5°F), and the normal axillary (skin) temperature 37·0°C (98·4°F). If the temperature is 0·5°C above these levels, the infant has a fever. In the prodromal period of any infectious disease of childhood, fever may be the only symptom.

Specific causes

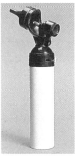

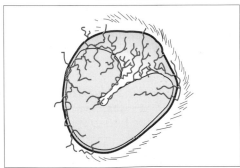

Tonsillitis—There may be small areas of pus on the tonsils or the throat may be generally red. The presence of pus does not help to distinguish between bacterial infection due to group A streptococcus (*Streptococcus pyogenes*) and a viral infection. Petechiae on the soft palate usually indicate a viral infection. A throat swab should be taken and a 10-day course of oral penicillin given.

Acute otitis media—An early sign is an increase in the size of the vessels of the upper posterior part of the drum. Later the drum becomes dull pink or red, and in severe cases there is bulging. Ear drums can be examined efficiently only if the auriscope has a magnifying lens. It is important to look for swelling or tenderness over the mastoids. The first choice of drugs is oral amoxycillin or erythromycin. If these are not effective, cefaclor or amoxycillin with clavulanic acid is given. The drum should be examined again after two days, and if there is no improvement the antibiotic should be changed.

Septicaemia—There are no specific signs. The infant appears extremely ill. In meningococcal septicaemia there is a generalised purpuric rash. Intravenous or intramuscular penicillin (300 mg) should be given immediately and the infant admitted, with the doctor taking the child to hospital personally if necessary. An infant with meningococcal septicaemia may die within a few hours of the onset of symptoms.

Meningitis—Irritability, drowsiness, and vomiting are common. A convulsion accompanied by fever may be the first sign. Neck stiffness is rare and raised anterior fontanelle tension is a late sign. Unusual drowsiness is a sinister symptom and the patient needs to be admitted for a lumbar puncture.

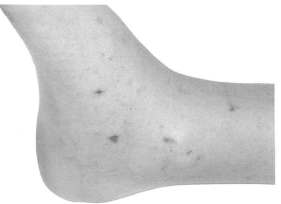

Meningococcal rash.

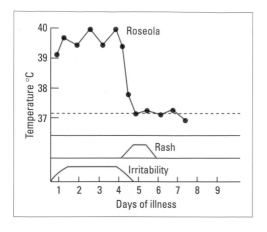

Roseola—Although fever may be present in the prodromal period of any infectious disease of childhood, pronounced fever is a notorious feature of roseola infantum. It usually occurs between 6 months and 3 years. The temperature usually reaches 39 to 40°C and remains at this level for about three days. The temperature falls as discrete minute pink macules appear on the trunk; these may spread to the limbs within a few hours. The infant appears less ill than might be expected from the height of the fever. The suboccipital, cervical, and postauricular lymph nodes are often enlarged and the blood picture frequently shows neutropenia.

Symptoms of urinary tract infection

- Fever
- Vomiting
- Lethargy
- Slow gain in weight

Urinary tract infection—Urinary tract infection in children often present simply with fever. It is essential that a carefully taken specimen of urine is sent to the laboratory promptly. The presence or absence of proteinuria is of no value in the diagnosis or exclusion of a urinary tract infection. Possibly the child may have to be admitted because an accurate diagnosis is essential. A course of trimethoprim is started, and the treatment can be changed the following day when the results of antibiotic sensitivity tests are received.

A clean catch urine specimen from an infant or a midstream urine specimen from an older child is the ideal. Only social cleanliness and dryness are required. If these techniques are not effective, a bag urine specimen should be obtained while the infant is held upright and the specimen transferred from the bag as soon as it is passed. A negative result from a bag urine specimen is reliable, but a positive result should be confirmed by a clean catch specimen or, in infants under 1 year old, by suprapubic puncture or, rarely, by a catheter specimen. If suprapubic aspiration is needed, the infant should be referred to hospital for day care or inpatient investigation.

The specimen of urine should ideally be collected in a sterile container, cooled immediately to 4°C, and examined in the laboratory within two hours. The method and time of collection must be stated on the pathology request to enable the microbiologist to give an accurate opinion. An alternative is to refrigerate the specimen at 4°C in the main compartment of a domestic refrigerator for, at most, 48 hours before examination. The temperature of the general practice refrigerator should be checked regularly. Another possibility is to transport the urine in 1·8% boric acid, but the correct amount of urine must be added to the bottle to ensure the correct concentration of boric acid.

The dipslide is a miniature culture plate that is immersed in the urine immediately after or during voiding. This eliminates the delay incurred during transport of the specimen to the laboratory.

Infants aged under 1 year should have an ultrasound examination of the renal tract, isotope renal scanning, cystourethrography, and plain abdominal radiography. Ultrasound examination and plain abdominal radiography are carried out during the acute phase, cystourethrography is performed when the urine is sterile, and isotope (^{99m}Tc dimercaptosuccinic acid (DMSA)) scanning is carried out three months after the acute phase. DMSA scanning detects scars, ultrasound examination shows obstructive lesions, and cystourethrography detects vesicoureteric reflux and should be performed under the protection of a suitable antibiotic.

Regular urine cultures are advisable at three monthly intervals as well as at times of fever or recurrence of symptoms. The urine should be cultured regularly while vesicoureteric reflux persists and in children with renal damage at least until the kidneys are fully grown (about the age of 16 years). The child's growth and blood pressure should be measured regularly.

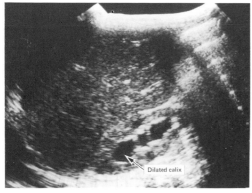

Ultrasound scan of kidney.

Fever in the older infant

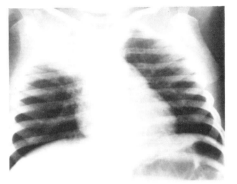

Radiograph showing pneumonia.

Pneumonia—A raised respiratory rate at rest and fever may be the only signs of pneumonia and a chest radiograph may be necessary to show consolidation. The upper limit for the normal respiratory rate is 60 per minute for infants less than 2 months of age, and 50 per minute between 2 and 12 months. Movements of the alae nasi and indrawing of the chest wall between the ribs are confirmatory signs.

Osteomyelitis or septic arthritis may present with fever. In the early stages the only helpful sign may be the infant's reluctance to move a limb, and radiographs are often normal. Later there is redness, swelling, and tenderness at the site of the osteomyelitis, which usually affects the maxilla, long bones, or vertebrae in infants. Early blood culture and radioisotope bone scans are helpful in the diagnosis.

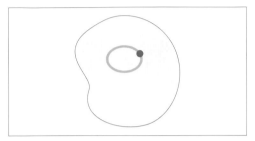

Malarial parasite in red cell.

Malaria—If within the previous two years the child has been in an area where malaria is endemic, blood films should be examined immediately for malarial parasites. The parasites are most numerous during fever but may be found at any time.

Pyrexia of undetermined origin

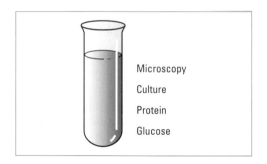

Microscopy
Culture
Protein
Glucose

Infants have no localising symptoms or signs. If they simply have fever, they should be seen again within a few hours or admitted to a cubicle on a children's ward for observation. Usually these children will have a full blood count, urine microscopy and culture, and sometimes blood culture and CSF examination.

CONVULSIONS IN THE OLDER INFANT

In infants between the ages of 1 month and 1 year convulsions are usually associated with fever. If there is no fever, epilepsy should be considered.

Fits can be divided into generalised or partial seizures. Generalised seizures include tonic-clonic and myoclonic fits. Partial seizures include focal motor and temporal lobe fits. During some episodes partial seizures may be followed by generalised seizures.

Generalised tonic-clonic fits are the most common type. The child may appear irritable or show other unusual behaviour for a few minutes before an attack. Sudden loss of consciousness occurs during the tonic phase, which lasts 20–30 seconds and is accompanied by temporary cessation of respiratory movements and central cyanosis. The clonic phase follows and there are jerky movements of the limbs and face. The movements gradually stop and the child may sleep for a few minutes before waking confused and irritable.

Although a typical tonic-clonic attack is easily recognised, other forms of fits may be difficult to diagnose from the mother's history. Infantile spasms may begin with momentary episodes of loss of tone, which can occur in bouts and be followed by fits in which the head may suddenly drop forward or the whole infant may move momentarily like a frog. Recurrent episodes with similar features, whether they are changes in the level of consciousness or involuntary movements, should raise the possibility of fits.

Tonic
- Cry
- Loss of consciousness
- Rigidity
- Apnoea

Clonic
- Repetitive limb movement (rate can be counted)

Sleep

Dangers

- Inhalation of vomit
- Hypoxaemia

Differential diagnosis

Convulsions must be differentiated from blue breath-holding attacks, which usually begin at 9 to 18 months. Immediately after a frustrating or painful experience infants cry vigorously and suddenly hold their breath, become cyanosed, and in the most severe cases lose consciousness. Rarely, their limbs become rigid, and there may be a few clonic movements lasting a few seconds. Respiratory movements begin again and infants gain consciousness immediately. The attacks diminish with age with no specific treatment. The mother may be helped to manage these extremely frightening episodes by being told that the child will not die and that she should handle each attack consistently by putting the child on his side.

Rigors may occur in any acute febrile illness, but there is no loss of consciousness.

Pain or frustration

? Breath holding attack

Febrile convulsions

A febrile convulsion is a fit occurring in a child aged from 6 months to 5 years, precipitated by fever arising from infection outside the nervous system in a child who is otherwise neurologically normal.

Convulsions with fever include any convulsion in a child of any age with fever of any cause. Among children who have convulsions with fever are those with pyogenic or viral meningitis, encephalitis, or cerebral palsy with intercurrent infections. Children who have a prolonged fit or who have not completely recovered within one hour should be suspected of having one of these conditions.

Most of the fits that occur between the ages of 6 months and 5 years are simple febrile convulsions and have an excellent prognosis.

By arbitrary definition, in simple febrile convulsions the fit lasts less than 20 minutes, there are no focal features, and the child is aged between 6 months and 5 years and has been developing normally.

Simple febrile convulsions

All the following:
- <20 minutes
- No focal features
- 6 months to 5 years
- No developmental or neurological abnormalities
- Not repeated in the same episode
- Complete recovery within one hour

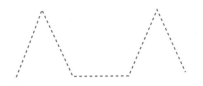

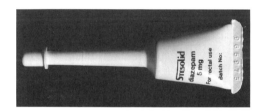

Often fever is recognised only when a convulsion has already occurred. Febrile convulsions are usually of the tonic-clonic type. The objective of emergency treatment is the prevention of a prolonged fit (lasting over 20 minutes), which may be followed by permanent brain damage, epilepsy, and developmental delay.

An electroencephalogram (EEG) is not a guide to diagnosis, treatment, or prognosis.

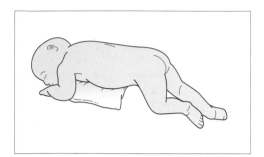

Emergency treatment

A child who has fever should have all his clothes removed and should be covered with a sheet only. He should be nursed on his side or prone with his head to one side because vomiting with aspiration is a constant hazard.

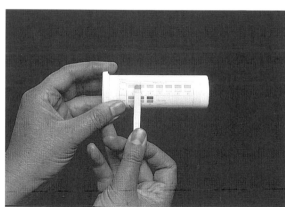

Rectal diazepam (0·5 mg/kg) produces an effective blood concentration of anticonvulsant within 10 minutes. The most convenient preparation resembles a toothpaste tube (Stesolid). Early admission to hospital or transfer to the intensive care unit should be considered if a second dose of anticonvulsant is needed.

All children who have had a first febrile convulsion should be admitted to hospital to exclude meningitis and to educate the parents, as many fear that their child is dying during the fit. Physical examination at this stage usually does not show a cause for the fever, but a specimen of urine should be examined in the laboratory to exclude infection and a BM stix test should be performed. Blood should be taken for blood culture and plasma glucose and calcium estimations. Most of these children have a generalised viral infection with viraemia. A febrile convulsion may occur in roseola at the onset and three days later the rash appears. Occasionally, acute otitis media is present, in which case an antibiotic is indicated, but most children with febrile convulsions do not need an antibiotic. A pupuric rash suggests meningococcal septicaemia and the need for penicillin to be given immediately either intravenously or intramuscularly (see page 80).

Lumbar puncture—A lumbar puncture should be performed if the child is under 18 months old or any of the following are present:
  (*a*) signs of meningism such as neck stiffness;
  (*b*) drowsiness, irritability, or systemic illness;
  (*c*) complex convulsion that contains *any* feature that does not conform with the definitions of a simple convulsion.
Ideally, the decision should be taken by an experienced doctor, who may decide on clinical grounds that lumbar puncture is unnecessary even in a younger child, but when in doubt the investigation should be performed. The doctor deciding not to undertake a lumbar puncture should review the patient personally within a few hours. Children less than 2 years of age may have meningitis with *no* neck stiffness or other specific signs.

A child who has had severe vomiting or is in coma must be examined by an experienced doctor before lumbar puncture because of the risk of coning.

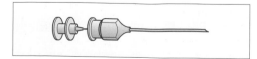

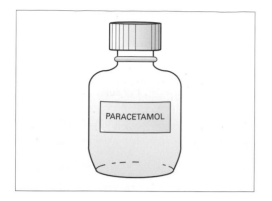

Management of fever—There is no evidence that antipyretic treatment influences the recurrence of febrile convulsions, but fever should be treated to promote the comfort of the child and to prevent dehydration. The child's clothes should be taken off and he should be covered with a sheet only. Paracetamol is the preferred antipyretic, and adequate fluid should be given.

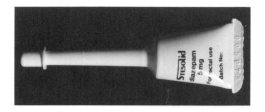

Anticonvulsant drugs—Rectal diazepam should be used as soon as possible after the onset of the convulsion. The parents should be advised not to give it if the convulsion has stopped.

The indications for long-term anticonvulsant prophylaxis have changed and the sole indication—frequent recurrences, which should be treated with phenobarbitone—is rare. There is no evidence that in the minority of children who later develop epilepsy the prophylactic use of anticonvulsant drugs would have prevented it.

Immunisation

As immunisation against diphtheria, tetanus, pertussis, and poliomyelitis is given to children 2–4 months old, this schedule is usually completed before febrile convulsions occur. Babies having convulsions with fever aged under 6 months should be assessed by a paediatrician. Children who have febrile convulsions before immunisation against diphtheria, pertussis, and tetanus because the immunisation has been delayed should be immunised after their parents have been instructed about the management of fever and the use of rectal diazepam.

Measles, mumps, and rubella immunisation should be given as usual to children who have had febrile convulsions, with advice about the management of fever to the parents. Rectal diazepam should be made available for use should a convulsion occur.

Prognosis

Unless there is clinical doubt about the child's current developmental or neurological state, parents should be told that prognosis for development is excellent. The risk of subsequent epilepsy after a single febrile convulsion with no complex features is about 1%. With each additional complex feature the risk rises to 13% in those children with two or more complex features. Only about 1% of children with febrile convulsions are in this group.

The risk of having further febrile convulsions is about 30%. This risk increases in younger infants and is about 50% in infants aged under 1 year at the time of their first convulsion. A history of febrile convulsions in a first-degree relative is also associated with a risk of recurrence of about 50%. A complex convulsion or a family history of epilepsy is probably associated with an increase in the risk of further febrile convulsions.

Information for parents

Information for parents should include:
- (*a*) an explanation of the nature of febrile convulsions, including information about the prevalence and prognosis;
- (*b*) instructions about the management of fever, the management of a convulsion, and the use of rectal diazepam;
- (*c*) reassurance.

This advice should be given verbally and a supplementary leaflet is helpful (see page 86).

Features of complex febrile convulsions:

- Lasting >20 minutes
- Focal
- More than one on the same day
- Developmental or neurological abnormalities

Advice to parents: Febrile convulsions

Your child has had a febrile convulsion. We know it was a very frightening experience for you. You may have thought that your child was dead or dying, as many parents think that when they first see a febrile convulsion. Febrile convulsions are not as serious as they appear.

What is a febrile convulsion?
It is an attack brought on by fever in a child aged between six months and five years.

What is a convulsion?
A convulsion is an attack in which the child becomes unconscious and usually stiff, with jerking of the arms and legs. It is caused by unusual electrical activity of the brain. The words convulsion, fit, and seizure have the same meaning.

What shall I do if my child has another convulsion?
Lay him on his side, with his head on the same level or slightly lower than the body. Note the time. Do not try to force anything into his mouth. Do not slap or shake the child.

The hospital may give you medicine to insert into your child's bottom. This is called rectal diazepam. If the convulsion has not stopped by the time that you have found the tube, insert it into the child's bottom and express the contents of the tube. This treatment should stop the convulsion within 10 minutes. If it does not, take your child to the hospital. You may need to dial 999 to obtain an ambulance. Let your doctor know what has happened.

About one child in 30 will have had a febrile convulsion by the age of five years.

Is it epilepsy?
No. The word epilepsy is applied to fits without fever, usually in older children and adults.

Do febrile convulsions lead to epilepsy?
Rarely; 99 out of 100 children with febrile convulsions never have convulsions after they reach school age, and never have fits without fever.

Do febrile convulsions cause permanent brain damage?
Almost never. Very rarely, a child who has a very prolonged febrile convulsion lasting half an hour or more may suffer permanent damage from it.

What starts febrile convulsions?
Any illness that causes a high temperature, usually a cold or other virus infection.

Will it happen again?
Three out of 10 children who have a febrile convulsion will have another one. The risk of having another febrile convulsion falls rapidly after the age of 3 years.

Does the child suffer discomfort or pain during a convulsion?
No. The child is unconscious and unaware of what is happening.

What shall I do if my child has fever?
You can take the child's temperature by placing the bulb of the thermometer under his armpit for three minutes with his arm held against his side. Keep him cool by taking off his clothes and reducing the room temperature. Give plenty of fluids to drink. Give children's paracetamol medicine to reduce the temperature. The following doses should be given:
  Up to 1 year old   one 5 ml spoonful (120 mg)
  Aged 1 to 3 years   two 5 ml spoonfuls (240 mg)
  Aged 4 years and over   three 5 ml spoonfuls (360 mg).
Repeat the dose every four hours until the temperature falls to normal, and then every six hours for the next 24 hours.

If the child seems ill or has ear ache or sore throat, let your doctor see him or her in case any other treatment, such as an antibiotic, is needed. Antibiotics are not necessary for most children with fever due to virus infections.

Is regular treatment with tablets or medicine necessary?
Usually not. The doctor will explain to you if your child needs regular medicine.

Adapted from a pamphlet produced by the British Paediatric Association

CRYING BABIES

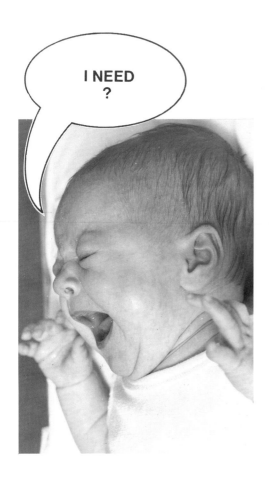

Apart from the subtle method of eye to eye communication, babies have no other way of signalling their needs to their mothers than by crying. Babies who are quiet or "good" may be abnormal or ill. As crying is a non-specific call for help, obvious needs should be investigated. In most cases no remediable cause is found and the problem may resolve spontaneously when infants are about 3 months old. By then, however, parents may have become exhausted from lack of sleep, and marital discord may follow while the infant remains fresh. As well as suggesting any appropriate management, the family doctor should encourage parents to take one or two evenings off together each week to visit friends or go to a film. Parents often worry that the infant is suffering from lack of sleep and wrongly ascribe poor appetite or frequent colds to this cause.

Sound spectrography has confirmed the clinical impression that cries of cerebral irritability, pain, and hunger are different in quality, but this method is not available to most clinicians. During the first month infants do not shed tears when they cry, and even after the age of about 6 months many infants cry at night without shedding tears.

The doctor needs to take a full history, including details of the pattern of crying, when the problem began, and measures taken to resolve it. It should be possible to determine whether the infant has always needed little sleep or whether he has developed a habit of crying in order to get into his parents' comfortable bed. The doctor should also explore the reason why the parents have sought advice at this stage. The mother should be asked about any change in the house, where the infant sleeps, and who looks after him during the day. Illnesses in the child or family and marital and social backgrounds also need considering. A physical examination usually shows no abnormality, but occasionally there may be signs of acute otitis media.

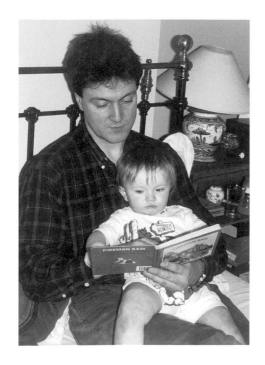

Difficulty in getting to sleep may be avoided by starting a bedtime ritual in infancy. A warm bath followed by being wrapped in particular blankets may later be replaced by the mother or father reading from a book or singing nursery rhymes before the light is turned out. A soft cuddly toy of any type can lie next to the infant from shortly after birth, and seeing this familiar toy again may help to induce sleep.

The parents should be told that during the night babies often open their eyes and move their limbs and heads. They should be asked to resist getting up to see their baby, as the noise of getting out of bed may wake him and he may then remain awake. Babies who do wake may be pacified with a drink and may then fall asleep. The drink is to provide comfort rather than to assuage any thirst.

Parents whose young children sleep a great deal during the day can discourage them from doing this by taking them out shopping or giving them other diversions, and they may then sleep well at night.

Sleep disturbance is a common reaction to the trauma of admission to hospital or moving house, and taking the child into the parents' room for a few weeks may help to reassure the infant that he has not been abandoned.

If the infant is prepared to go to sleep at a certain time but the parents would like to advance it by an hour, they can put him to bed five minutes earlier each night until the planned bedtime is achieved.

Hunger and thirst

Babies often cry and become restless just before a feed is due, and in the early weeks of life the infant may demand to be fed three hourly or even two hourly. This is perfectly normal. Preterm infants need particularly high milk intakes for "catch up" growth and they may become less demanding when they reached their final centiles for weight.

The volumes of bottled milk recommended are only average amounts, and many infants will therefore need more to prevent excessive hunger. Regular weighing and use of a growth chart to plot the results are the only ways of ensuring that the infant is obtaining the correct amount of feeds. Feeding at regular intervals is apt to cause crying in many babies, and demand feeding is preferable. Some infants scream when they approach the breast, and the help of an experienced midwife is needed to overcome this problem.

The age at which infants sleep through the night and do not require a night feed varies greatly. It usually occurs when infants weigh about 5 kg, and parents may be worried because their neighbour's child of a similar age has already omitted the night feed. Similar competition between mothers over which baby first manages three meals a day may also lead to inadequate feeding, followed by crying.

It is impossible to determine the difference between a cry due to hunger and a cry due to thirst. The only way of solving this problem is to offer infants water twice daily. This can easily be given mid-morning or mid-afternoon. Some infants dislike the taste of boiled tap water so a little fruit juice or half a teaspoon of sugar can be added to 100 ml (4 floz) of water.

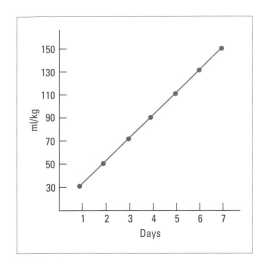

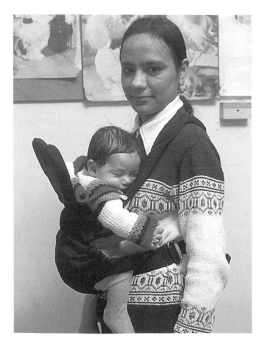

Even newborn infants cry to obtain physical contact and the crying stops as soon as they are picked up. It does not spoil babies to pick them up when they want contact. Once they are a few weeks old infants begin to have periods of waking, and some will not tolerate being left in a pram or cot by themselves. A harness that allows them to remain in contact with their mother's body will often satisfy these infants. Alternatively, a canvas chair can be used even as early as 1 month, and can be placed in a safe position in the kitchen or wherever the mother is working.

If babies do not stop crying when held, walking with them, rocking them, or taking them for a car ride may stop the crying.

Wrapping infants in a blanket and putting them firmly into a carrycot or a very small cot may also provide contact, although by an impersonal method.

Non-nutritive sucking stops crying, provided babies are not hungry. Putting a dummy into the mouth of a crying baby who is not hungry may be effective as a temporary measure.

Three months' colic and feeding problems

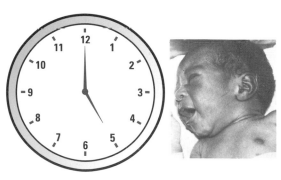

Three months' colic is the name given to a syndrome that usually begins at about 2 weeks of age and has usually stopped by 4 months. The infant screams, draws up his legs, and cannot be comforted by milk, being picked up, or having his napkin changed. This usually occurs in the early evening, when the mother is busy getting supper ready, has less time to play with the baby, and may be anxious. Breast feeding mothers may have less milk at that time of the day.

Some babies swallow excessive air during feeding as a result of milk spurting from the breast or a very small hole in the teat of the bottle. Mothers usually complain that these infants gulp at the beginning of the feed and they have particular difficulty in bringing up the wind. This problem does not occur in societies where babies are held on the

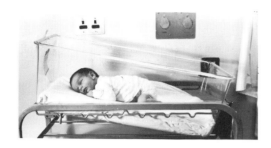

mothers' backs for most of the day. The infant's abdomen is pressed against the mother's back and the infant is kept upright, which is the best position for releasing excessive gastric air.

If the milk spurts from the breast, the first 25 ml (1 floz) or so should be expressed manually and given to the infant later if necessary. If the baby is fed by bottle, the size of the hole in the bottle teat should be checked and made larger with a hot needle if necessary. The infant can be winded most easily by putting him prone with his head higher than his feet, but he must be observed constantly while in this position.

Other causes

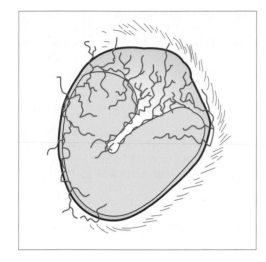

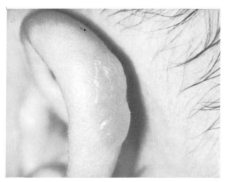

Non-accidental injury to pinna.

Illness—If the infant starts crying persistently, especially if he has not cried like this before, disease should be suspected. Acute otitis media often causes persistent crying at night, but meningitis or a urinary tract infection may have no specific signs. An intussusception is an invagination of a proximal part of the gut into a more distal portion and may result in partial or complete intestinal obstruction. The infant has sudden attacks of screaming and pallor that last for a few minutes and recur every 10 to 20 minutes. Between attacks the infant appears normal. Blood stained mucus may be passed rectally. The abdomen is tender only during attacks, but often there is a mass over the course of the colon. If intussusception is suspected the infant should be admitted to hospital (see p 52).

Mechanical problems—Babies do not seem distressed when their napkins are wet or soiled, though some cry when they are being undressed or changed. An open safety pin is an extremely rare cause of crying.

Fatigue—When young infants have been on a long journey or have been stimulated more than usual by playing with relatives, they may become irritable and not keen to sleep.

Failure of mother–infant adjustment—Crying may be a sign of this failure, which may be related to the character of the infant as much as the response of the mother. The crying may represent the difficulties of each adjusting to the other. If an infant has been crying persistently for several weeks the possibility of severe depression in the mother should be considered. This depression could be the cause or the result of the crying. The mother is exhausted by lack of sleep and particularly liable to injure her infant, and both mother and infant may need to be admitted to hospital for diagnosis and management.

For most infants none of the above reasons for crying are present. The parents need reassuring strongly after examination that their infant is healthy and that the problem will resolve spontaneously. Sedation of the infant with chloral hydrate for a week during a difficult period may enable the mother to regain some of her strength. The drug should not be used for longer, since it loses its effect. Only a few doses should be prescribed, as the mother may take them herself or give too many to her infant in a depressive episode.

Special problems after the age of 3 months

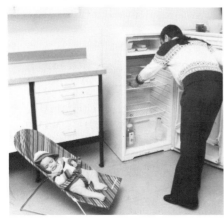

Loneliness is probably the commonest cause of crying after the age of 3 months. While they are awake during the day some infants will not tolerate being left alone but are happy if they are left in the room where the mother is working. These infants are extremely interested in their surroundings and need the stimulation of things going on around them. Similarly, infants need to be propped up when out in their prams, and when they begin to reach out they need simple toys to play with.

Separation from the mother during admission to hospital or when parents go on holiday by themselves may be followed by bouts of crying. An infant can relate to only two or three adults at a time, and frequent changes in caretaker may be associated with crying.

After about 5 months infants may cry when a stranger approaches them or when they sleep in a different room. They may wake suddenly and appear terrified, which might be due to a nightmare, although there is no method of proving this.

Crying babies

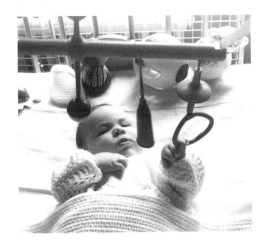

Infants who do not sleep after 3 months

During the first few weeks of life some babies sleep almost continuously for the 24 hours whereas others sleep for only about 12 hours. Many mothers consider that a new born baby should sleep continuously and do not realise that babies take an interest in what is going on around them. Infants who need little sleep may wake regularly at 2 or 4 am and remain awake for two or three hours. Some are settled by a drink, but others cry persistently after this and the mother may take the infant into her own bed before they go to sleep. Some infants wake in a similar way but are then content to remain awake looking at mobiles above their cots or playing with toys left in the cot.

Behaviour modification and drugs

Mon	Sleep		Nap	Sleep	

Shade in the times your child is asleep   Leave blank the times your child is awake

	Midnight 12	2	4	6	8	10	Noon 12	2	4	6	8	10	Midnight 12
Mon													
Tue													
Wed													
Thur													
Fri													
Sat													
Sun													

When infants wake frequently during the night and cry persistently until they are taken into their parents' bed, a plan of action is needed. If there is an obvious cause, such as acute illness or recent admission to hospital, the problem may resolve itself within a few weeks, and at first there need be no change in management. If there is no obvious cause, the parents are asked to keep a record of the infant's sleep pattern for two weeks (see sleep history chart). This helps to determine where the main problem lies and can be used as a comparison with treatment.

Both parents are seen at the next visit; both need to accept that they must be firm and follow the plan exactly. Behaviour modification is the only method that produces long-term improvement, but it can be combined with drugs initially if the mother is at breaking point.

Day	Time to bed	Time to sleep	First problem	What did you do?	Second problem	What did you do?	Time woke up in morning
Mon							
Tue							
Wed							
Thur							
Fri							
Sat							
Sun							

Behaviour modification separates the mother from the child gradually or abruptly, depending on the parents' and doctor's philosophy. The slow method starts with the mother giving a drink and staying with the child for decreasing lengths of time. In the next stage no drink is given. Then she speaks to the child through the closed door and, finally, does not go to the child at all. The abrupt method consists of letting the child cry it out; he stops after three or four nights. There are an infinite number of variations between these extremes, and the temperament of the parents, child, and doctor will determine what is acceptable.

Number of minutes to wait before going into your child briefly

| Day | At first episode | If your child is still crying | | |
		Second episode	Third episode	Subsequent episodes
1	5	10	15	15
2	10	15	20	20
3	15	20	25	25
4	20	25	30	30
5	25	30	35	35

Another approach is to increase the waiting time before going to the infant. In severe cases a written programme of several small changes can be given to the mother and she can be seen again by the health visitor or family doctor after each step has been achieved. The mother will need to be reassured that the infant will not develop a hernia from crying or vomit or choke, and neighbours may be pacified by being told that the child will soon be cured.

Many sleep problems can be resolved without drugs, but some mothers are so exhausted by loss of sleep that they cannot manage a programme of behaviour modification unless the infant receives some preliminary sedation. The most satisfactory drug for this age group is chloral hydrate 30 mg/kg body weight given one hour before going to bed. The full dose is given for two weeks, followed by a half dose for a week; the drug is then given on alternate nights for a week. The objective is to change the pattern of sleeping. A behaviour modification plan is needed during the third and subsequent weeks.

WHOOPING COUGH

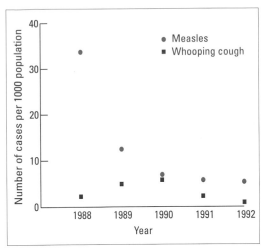

Source: OPCS

Young infants receive no protective immunity to whooping cough from their mothers and have the highest incidence of complications. Immunisation is directed at increasing herd immunity and reducing the exposure of infants to older children who have the disease. Recent changes in advice on contraindications to whooping cough vaccine have been associated with the increased use of this vaccine.

Contraindications to immunisation

> Is the baby unwell in any way? YES/NO
>
> Has the baby had any side effects from previous immunisation? YES/NO
>
> Did the baby behave normally during the first week of life? YES/NO
>
> Has the baby, or anyone in the immediate family, ever had fits or convulsions? YES/NO
>
> Is the baby developing normally? YES/NO

Mothers can fill out a card in the waiting room at each visit for immunisation.

Post-immunisation fever

The doctor should advise the parent that if fever develops after immunisation the child may be given a dose of paracetamol followed, if necessary, by a second dose 4–6 hours later. The dose of paracetamol for post-immunisation fever for an infant aged 2–3 months is 60 mg; an oral syringe can be obtained from any pharmacy to give the small volume required. The doctor should warn the parent that medical advice should be sought if the fever persists after the second dose.

Convulsions and encephalopathy have been reported as rare complications, but these conditions may arise from other causes and be falsely attributed to the vaccine. Neurological complications after whooping cough itself are considerably more common than after the vaccine.

As with any other elective immunisation procedure, if a child is suffering from any acute illness then vaccination should be postponed until the child has fully recovered. Minor infections without fever or systemic upset, however, are not reasons to delay immunisation. Vaccination should not be carried out in children who have a history of a severe local or general reaction to a preceding dose; the following reactions should be regarded as severe:

Local—an extensive area of redness and swelling, which becomes indurated and covers most of the antero-lateral surface of the thigh or a major part of the circumference of the upper arm.

General—fever (a temperature of 39·5°C or higher) within 48 hours of vaccination, anaphylaxis, bronchospasm, laryngeal oedema, generalised collapse, prolonged unresponsiveness, prolonged inconsolable screaming, and convulsions occurring within 72 hours.

A personal or family history of allergy is *not* a contraindication to immunisation against whooping cough; nor are stable neurological conditions such as cerebral palsy or spina bifida.

Children with problem histories

When there is a personal or family history of *febrile* convulsions then there is an increased risk of these occurring after pertussis immunisation. In such children immunisation is *recommended*, but advice on the *prevention of fever* (see box) should be given at the time of immunisation.

In a recent British study, children with a family history of epilepsy were immunised with pertussis vaccine without any appreciable adverse events. These children's developmental progress has been normal. In children who have a close (first degree) relative with *idiopathic epilepsy* there may be a risk of developing a similar condition, irrespective of whether they are vaccinated. Immunisation is *recommended* for these children.

When there is a *still evolving neurological problem* immunisation should be *deferred* until the condition is stable. When there has been a documented history of *cerebral damage in the neonatal period* immunisation *should be carried out unless there is evidence of an evolving neurological abnormality.* If immunisation is to be deferred, this should be stated on the neonatal discharge summary. When there is doubt, appropriate advice should be sought from a consultant paediatrician, district immunisation coordinator, or consultant in public health medicine *rather than withholding the vaccine.*

Diagnosis

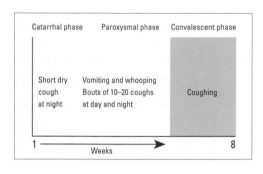

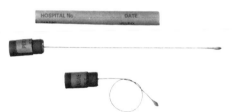

Whooping cough is difficult to diagnose during the first 7–14 days of the illness (catarrhal phase), when there is a short dry cough at night. Later, bouts of 10–20 short dry coughs occur day and night; each is on the same high note or rises in pitch. A long attack of coughing is followed by a sharp indrawing of breath, which may produce the crowing sound, or whoop. Some children, especially babies, with *Bordetella pertussis* infection never develop the whoop. Feeding with crumbly food often provokes a coughing spasm, which may culminate in vomiting. Afterwards there is a short period when the child can be fed again without provoking coughing. In uncomplicated cases there are no abnormal respiratory signs.

The most important differential diagnosis in infants is bronchiolitis; this is usually due to the respiratory syncytial virus, which produces epidemics of winter cough in infants under 1 year. For the first few days there may be only bouts of vibratory rasping cough, which never produce a whoop. Later, rhonchi or crepitations are heard in the chest and the infant either deteriorates or improves rapidly within a few days. Older siblings infected with the virus may have a milder illness. Other viruses may cause acute bronchitis with coughing but there are seldom more than two coughs at a time.

A properly taken pernasal swab plated promptly on a specific medium should reveal *B pertussis* in most patients during the first few weeks of the illness. A blood lymphocyte count of $10 \times 10^9/l$ or more with normal erythrocyte sedimentation rate suggests whooping cough.

Management

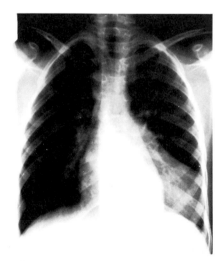

Normal radiograph.

If the diagnosis is suspected in the catarrhal phase (usually because a sibling has had recognisable whooping cough) a 10-day course of erythromycin may be given to the child and to other children in the home. Parents must be warned that an antibiotic may shorten the course of the disease only in the early stages and is unlikely to affect established illness. Vomiting can be treated by giving soft, not crumbly, food or small amounts of fluid hourly.

No medicine reliably reduces the cough. Salbutamol has been used in a dosage of 0·3 mg/kg/24 hours divided into three doses, When sleep is disturbed some authorities recommend that the child should be given a bedtime dose of 3–5 mg/kg of phenobarbitone. In severe cases mothers can be taught to give physiotherapy, which may help to clear secretions, especially before the infant goes to sleep. An attack may be stopped by a gentle slap on the back.

The threshold for admission to hospital should be lower for children aged under 6 months. Convulsions and cyanosis during coughing attacks are absolute indications for admission to an isolation cubicle. Parents often become exhausted by sleep loss, and arranging for different members of the family to sleep with the child will give the mother a respite. The cough usually lasts for 8 to 12 weeks and may recur when the child has any new viral respiratory infection during the subsequent year. If the child is generally ill or the cough has not improved after six weeks, a chest radiograph should be performed to exclude bronchopneumonia or lobar collapse, which need treatment with physiotherapy and antibiotics. Long-term effects on the lung, such as bronchiectasis, are rare in developed countries.

The infant will not be infective for other children after about four weeks from the beginning of the illness or about two days after erythromycin is started. The incubation period is about seven days, and contacts who have no symptoms two weeks after exposure have usually escaped infection.

USEFUL INFORMATION

Circumcision and undescended testis

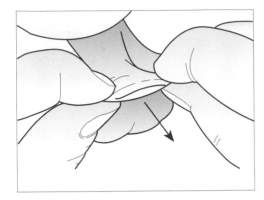

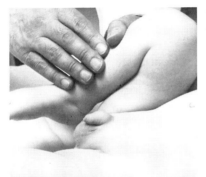

In 95% of babies the foreskin and glans of the penis are still united at birth. It has been found that the foreskin can be retracted by the age of 1 year in about half the babies and by the age of 3 years in nine out of ten. But no attempt should be made to retract the foreskin until the baby is about 4 years old. Attempts to retract the foreskin earlier are likely to injure the mucosa, causing bleeding followed by adhesions, and circumcision may later become necessary. Mothers often request circumcision to be carried out because the prepucial orifice appears small. In most cases the adequacy of the orifice can be shown by gently stretching the foreskin *distally* and no attempt should be made to retract the foreskin. Before the age of 4 years the only medical indications for circumcision are recurrent purulent balanitis and ballooning of the foreskin at the beginning of micturition.

Most circumcisions are performed as a religious ritual, in Jewish families on the 8th day of life and in Muslim boys between the ages of 3 and 15 years.

Spontaneous primary descent of the testes rarely occurs after the age of 4 months and never after 1 year. After the neonatal period an active cremasteric reflex can easily pull the testis out of the scrotum, especially if the examiner's hands are cold. The mother will often have noted whether the testes are both in the scrotum after a hot bath, and a retractile testis will descend into the scrotum when the thigh and knee are maximally flexed on that side. (See also page 23.)

Common napkin rashes

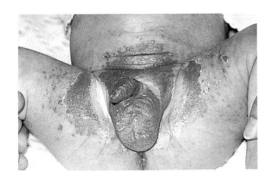

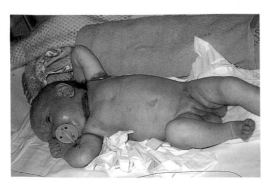
Seborrhoeic dermatitis.

Napkin rashes are usually due to ammoniacal dermatitis, seborrhoeic dermatitis, or perianal excoriation.

Ammoniacal dermatitis is caused by ammonia produced by faecal bacterial enzymes acting on urea in the urine. Erythema, papules, scaling, and erosions appear in areas that have been in contact with napkins soaked with urine. The depths of the skinfolds are spared and the prepuce and scrotum are especially vulnerable. The principle of treatment is to keep urine and faeces away from the skin. Initial treatment includes changing napkins frequently or leaving the child without a napkin. A zinc cream is applied to the affected area every time the napkin is changed; in resistant cases a silicone cream is used. Some authorities consider that the formation of ammonia does not play a major part in this condition and they prefer the term "irritant napkin dermatitis".

If the rash does not improve within 10 days *Candida* infection of the lesions should be considered. This rash has a fiery red appearance with a scaly edge, often with a few early papules separated from the main eruption. Nystatin cream should be applied to the rash each time the napkin is changed for at least a week. The infant's mouth should be examined to determine whether white plaques of *Candida* are present and an oral suspension of nystatin is needed. Alternatively, miconazole oral gel may be used. In breast fed infants the mother's nipples should be examined, as a scaling dermatitis of the nipples can be due to *Candida* and may reinfect the infant.

Any infant with a rash in the napkin area should be undressed completely to ensure that he or she does not have a rash elsewhere. In *seborrhoeic dermatitis* the erythema and scaling may also affect the axillae, neck, the area behind the ears, scalp, forehead, and eyelids. The scalp may be covered with adherent hard crusted plaques (cradle

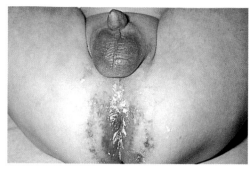

Perianal excoriation.

cap). Secondary infection by staphylococci, streptococci, or *Candida* is common. The condition always begins before the age of 3 months and clears completely without treatment by 9 months. In contrast to the infant with ammoniacal dermatitis, the infant with seborrhoeic dermatitis is oblivious of the rash. The cause is unknown and there is usually no family history of dermatitis. Treatment with 0·5% or 1% hydrocortisone ointment is rapidly effective and the lesions usually clear completely within a few weeks. In severe cases nystatin or an antibacterial agent may be added to the cream. Cradle cap can be removed by applying an ointment containing 0·5% salicyclic acid in soft paraffin for a week. It should be left on the scalp for about an hour once a day and then removed with shampoo.

If the rash affects mainly the perianal area, it is probably due to persistently loose stools. *Perianal excoriation* is commonly found in infants with gastroenteritis and resolves when the diarrhoea stops. Zinc cream or exposure may hasten the resolution of the lesions, but changes in the stool pH and consistency are the most important factors.

Sleeping position of infants

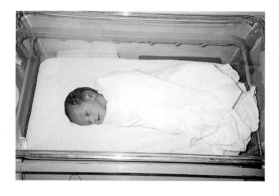

In November 1991 the Department of Health issued recommendations on the sleeping position of infants to try to reduce the incidence of cot death (Sudden Infant Death Syndrome). This followed assessment of several studies conducted around the world.

Babies should no longer be placed prone (on their front) when they are laid down to sleep. They should be placed either on their back (supine) or on their sides. Despite previous teaching, there is no evidence that placing healthy babies on their back results in an increased risk of death from choking or vomiting. There are, however, certain circumstances in which the babies should be nursed prone. These include some babies in neonatal units, babies with severe gastro-oesophageal reflux, babies receiving treatment in splints for unstable hips, and babies with Pierre Robin syndrome.

By 6–7 months of age, many babies will roll themselves over onto their front during sleep. There is no need for concern over this, as the incidence of cot death is markedly reduced by this age.

Cot deaths

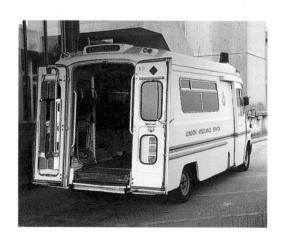

The Foundation for the Study of Infant Deaths (35 Belgrave Square, London SW1X 8PS, telephone 0171-235 1721) produces a leaflet on cot death for parents, which they may find helpful.

About one baby in every 1200 born alive dies suddenly and unexpectedly between the ages of 1 week and 2 years. Typically, an apparently healthy baby (or, occasionally, one with only minor symptoms) is put in a cot to rest and some time later is found dead. Although an infant may be face down in the cot with the bedclothes over him or her, suffocation should not be assumed. Sometimes vomit, which may be blood tinged, is found around the mouth or on the bedding, but regurgitation usually occurs after death and is not the cause of death.

In some cases necropsy discloses an unsuspected congenital abnormality or rapidly fatal infection. But usually there is no evidence of severe disease, though there might be slight reddening of the tracheal mucosa, which in other babies normally resolves spontaneously.

Parents often blame themselves and may worry that the infant suffocated as a result of neglect. They should be told that their feelings of guilt are a natural reaction, and the doctor should explain to them, and to anyone who was looking after the baby when death occurred, that cot death is a well recognised but ill-understood condition and that no one is to blame for the infant's death.

Parents must also be told that because the death is of unknown cause the coroner will have to be told as a matter of routine and that there will be a necropsy. If the parents want to see the infant's body (and they should be asked), the infant is clothed and a doctor or nurse should be present to answer questions and provide support. Discussion with the parents will determine who is best to help with their grieving.

The family doctor and health visitor should be informed of the death immediately. A child psychiatrist may be needed in the management of brothers and sisters. The family doctor should explain the results of the necropsy to the parents or arrange for a paediatrician to do this.

Equipment for examining children

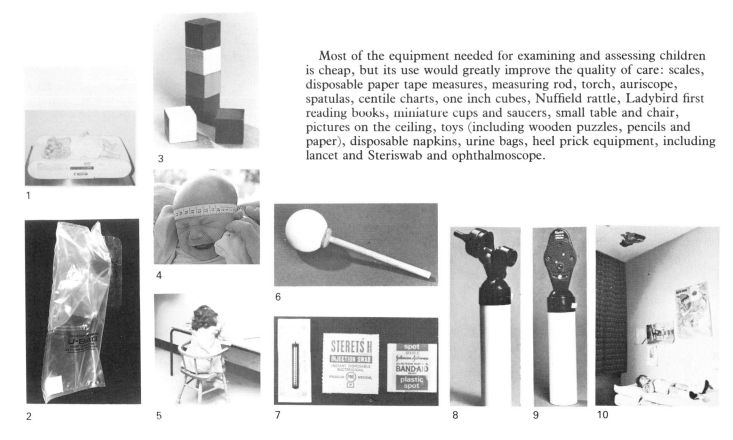

Most of the equipment needed for examining and assessing children is cheap, but its use would greatly improve the quality of care: scales, disposable paper tape measures, measuring rod, torch, auriscope, spatulas, centile charts, one inch cubes, Nuffield rattle, Ladybird first reading books, miniature cups and saucers, small table and chair, pictures on the ceiling, toys (including wooden puzzles, pencils and paper), disposable napkins, urine bags, heel prick equipment, including lancet and Steriswab and ophthalmoscope.

Essential equipment: (1) scales, (2) urine bag, (3) building blocks, (4) disposable paper tape, (5) small table and chair, (6) Nuffield rattle, (7) heel prick equipment, (8) auriscope, (9) ophthalmoscope, (10) pictures on the ceiling.

Examining an ill child

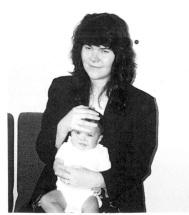

Throat examination.

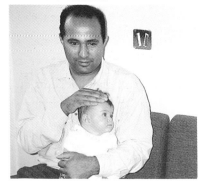

Ear examination.

Infants should be allowed to adopt whatever position they like (usually on their mother's knee) where they can be observed. The history taken from the mother must contain enough detail to provide a differential diagnosis before the physical examination begins.

A systematic examination may prove impossible in a protesting infant, so the most relevant system should be examined first. If the infant objects to being fully undressed, only the part being examined need be exposed. The examiner needs warm hands and should talk to the infant continuously to soothe him. Patience and gentleness at this stage are often rewarded by the infant accepting a full examination without protest.

The baby's abdomen is best examined as the infant lies on his mother's knees during a feed. Abdominal breathing is normal, and the edge of the liver is easily palpable. Even the newborn will show abdominal tenderness by grimacing or crying. Rectal examination may be performed with the little finger.

Instruments such as auriscopes and stethoscopes should be shown to the infant first and rested on his forearm so that he can see what they are. The auriscope must be used gently and the speculum not pushed too far into the external meatus. When the pinna is pulled gently outwards and downwwards, the tympanic membrane can be seen with the tip of the speculum in the outer end of the meatus.

Examination of the throat, which is the most disliked procedure, should be left until last. It should never be performed in an infant with stridor unless the examiner has the facilities to intubate the infant immediately.

The infant should be examined *again* no longer than 24 hours later, and the initiative for this review should not be left to the parents, who may not appreciate the danger of features that have developed.

Non-accidental injury

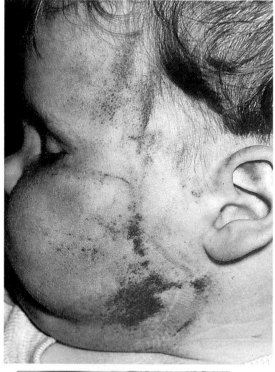

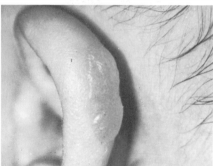

This section has been restricted to physical abuse, as sexual abuse is rare in infants less than a year of age.

Non-accidental injury inflicted by adults on children is often hard to detect. Symptoms that are difficult to explain may be the result of inflicted injury. In Britain as many as 100 children a year may die from non-accidental injuries.

Non-accidental injury should be suspected, especially in a child aged under 3, whenever: (a) there has been a delay between the accident occurring and the parents seeking medical help; (b) the explanation of the injury is inadequate, discrepant, or too plausible; (c) the child or sibling has a history of non-accidental or suspicious injury; (d) there is evidence of earlier injury; (e) the child has often been brought to the family doctor or accident department for little apparent reason; (f) the parents show disturbed behaviour or unusual reactions to the child's injuries or have a history of psychiatric illness; (g) the child shows obvious neglect or failure to thrive.

Typical initial injuries are: (a) burns, abrasions, or small bruises on the face; (b) injuries to the mouth or torn fraenulum of the tongue; (c) bruises caused by shaking or rough handling, including finger-shaped bruises; (d) subconjunctival or retinal haemorrhages. If the doctor suspects non-accidental injury, the child should be undressed completely and examined fully, with all signs of injury noted. If the doctor's suspicions are not allayed, he or she should ensure the immediate examination of the child by a consultant paediatrician. The family doctor should, if possible, not mention any suspicions to the parents, as they may refuse to allow this examination and it may impair his relationship with them.

If parents refuse to allow their child to be seen or want to remove the child from hospital too soon, the social services department, the police or National Society for the Prevention of Cruelty to Children may seek an emergency protection order, which allows the child to be kept in hospital for 8 days.

Children with genuinely accidental injuries will occasionally be admitted unnecessarily, but this should not deter any doctor from admitting a child when there is reasonable doubt about the cause of an injury.

Preventable causes of death

- Digoxin
- Penicillin intrathecally
- Chloramphenicol
- Glucose >20%
- Sodium bicarbonate >2·1%
- Potassium chloride solution

Six preparations of drugs are especially associated with avoidable deaths in children.

Ampoules of digoxin for use in adults should never be supplied to children's wards. Ampoules of digoxin made especially for children ensure that a fatal overdose cannot be given.

Penicillin given intrathecally has no therapeutic value. Errors are often made in dispensing the correct dose of penicillin for intrathecal use, with fatal results. This route should therefore never be used for penicillin.

Excessive doses of chloramphenicol can easily be given if the special infant preparation is not used.

Intravenous glucose solution should never be given at a concentration higher than 20%. Sodium bicarbonate solution should never be given intravenously at a concentration higher than 2·1%. Higher concentrations of either of these solutions are severely hypertonic and may be followed by sudden death or permanent brain damage.

A bag of intravenous fluid to which a potassium chloride solution has been added should be shaken thoroughly to avoid giving a bolus of potassium chloride solution, which may cause a fatal arrhythmia.

Selected drugs in the newborn

Intestinal absorption is variable and regurgitation of antibiotics common, so the intramuscular or intravenous route should usually be used initially. Intramuscular injections are given into the upper lateral

Useful information

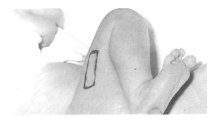

Intramuscular injection site.

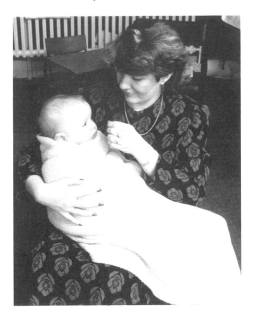

aspect of the thigh. Schemes for rotation of sites are essential to prevent local necrosis and to avoid further injections being given into a relatively avascular area. Drugs are usually given intramuscularly or orally every eight hours and intravenously by slow bolus injection every four or six hours. In preterm infants an adjustment of dose and frequency of administration may be needed and specific texts should be consulted.

Amoxycillin	(oral, IM, or IV)	50 mg/kg/24 h
Ampicillin	(oral, IM, or IV)	100 mg/kg/24 h
Ceftazidime	(IM or IV)	25–60 mg/kg/24 h
Chloral hydrate	(oral)	30–50 mg/kg per dose
Diazepam	(IM or IV)	200–300 microgram/kg per dose
Flucloxacillin	(oral, IM, or IV)	50 mg/kg/24 h
Gentamicin	(IM or IV)	5 mg/kg/24 h (12 hourly). Blood concentration *must* be checked
Miconazole gel	(oral)	2·5 ml twice daily
Naloxone	(IM or IV)	10–20 microgram/kg per dose
Nystatin	(oral)	100 000 units/dose (after feeds)
Paraldehyde	(IM)	0·1–0·2 ml/kg per dose
Benzylpenicillin	(IM or IV)	150 mg/kg/24 h
Phenobarbitone	(IM or IV)	15 mg/kg once only followed by 3 mg/kg per dose 12 hourly
Phenytoin	(IV)	15 mg/kg per dose slowly once followed by 3 mg/kg per dose 12 hourly
	(oral)	5 mg/kg/24 h
Sodium ironedetate	(oral)	1 ml twice daily
Triclofos	(oral)	50 mg/kg per dose

Some useful drugs in older infants

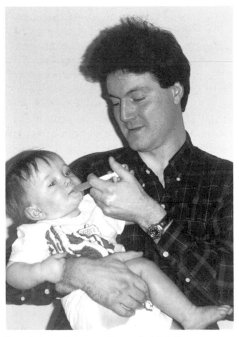

Special medicine syringes (which have no needles) can be used to measure and give small volumes accurately.

Infants treated at home and most of those in hospital need oral drugs three times a day. The drugs should be given before feeds and the infant need not be woken specially for them. Some preparations, particularly the penicillins, have an unpleasant taste and the medicine should not be mixed with food as the infant may then hate both. Syrup, which is a sucrose solution that forms the base of most elixirs, may cause dental caries if it is given regularly for a long time. If only one adult is present to give the medicine, wrapping the infant securely in a blanket may prevent spillage.

Amoxycillin   50 mg/kg/24 h
Ampicillin   100 mg/kg/24 h
Betamethasone   3 mg per dose intramuscularly or intravenously = 100 mg hydrocortisone
Cefaclor   60 mg/kg/24 h
Cefotaxime   100 mg/kg/24 h intramuscularly or intravenously (12 hourly)
Chloral hydrate   30–50 mg/kg/per dose
Co-trimoxazole   6 mg/kg/24 h (as trimethoprim)
Diazepam   200–300 microgram/kg orally per dose or slowly intravenously
Erythromycin   50 mg/kg/24 h
Flucloxacillin   50 mg/kg/24 h
Gentamicin   7 mg/kg/24 h intramuscularly or intravenously
Hydrocortisone   100 mg per dose intramuscularly or intravenously
Nystatin   100 000 units per dose (four hourly)
Paracetamol   75 mg/kg/24 h
Paraldehyde   0·15 ml/kg per dose intramuscularly
Benzylpenicillin   (intramuscularly or intravenously) 150 mg/kg/24 h
Phenoxymethylpenicillin   60 mg/kg/24 h
Phenobarbitone   5 mg/kg/24 h
Phenytoin   5 mg/kg/24 h
Trimeprazine tartrate   3 mg/kg per dose once daily

Special medicine syringes (which have no needles) can be used to measure and give small volumes accurately.

Taking blood

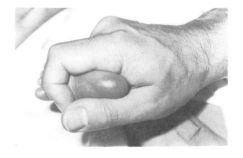

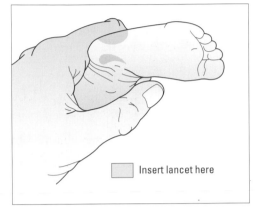

Insert lancet here

Capillary blood taken from infants aged up to 2 years can be used for a variety of tests. The commonest is the Guthrie test, but capillary blood may also be used for BM stix testing, haemoglobin estimations, and most biochemical tests.

The best site for taking capillary blood from an infant aged under 6 months is the heel. In older infants the thumb is a better site. The heel must be warm. If it is cold, the infant's foot should be dipped into hand hot water (40°C) for five minutes and dried thoroughly. The examiner then holds the infant's foot by encircling the ball of the heel with thumb and forefinger. The site selected for the heel prick must be on the side of the heel; if the ball or back of the heel is used a painful ulcer may form.

The site is wiped with ispropyl alcohol and allowed to dry. A disposable lancet is inserted into the heel about 2 mm and then withdrawn. Alternatively, a spring loaded lancet introducer may be used.

The initial drop of blood should be wiped away with a dry cotton swab and succeeding drops allowed to drip into the container on to the Guthrie test card, or on to the end of a BM stix. To milk blood into the heel the examiner should squeeze and release [his fingers] around the infant's calf and keep the heel below the rest of the leg. Up to 2 ml of blood can be obtained. When the required volume has been obtained, the heel is wiped and the wound pressed with a clean cotton wool ball. A small plaster should then be applied.

Teeth and teething

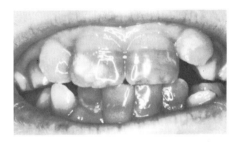

Severe discoloration due to tetracycline.

Although mothers consider that the eruption of the first tooth is a milestone in development, the age at which this occurs is of no practical importance. The first teeth to appear, at 6–12 months, are the lower incisors.

From the age of a few weeks infants normally put their fingers, and later anything else that comes to hand, into their mouths and mothers often wrongly ascribe this to teething.

Teething produces only teeth. It does not, contrary to common belief, cause convulsions, bronchitis, or napkin rash. Some mothers insist their infants are particularly irritable when they are teething, but it is important to examine the infant to exclude disease such as otitis media or meningitis before accepting the mother's explanation.

Dummies temporarily affect the growth of the mouth but there are no objections to using them. They should not be dipped in honey. Severe dental caries also follows the use of "comforters" or "dinky-feeders", which are filled with fluid containing sugar.

Tetracycline or its derivatives should never be given to children less than 8 years of age, as permanent brownish yellow staining of the teeth may occur.

Watering eye

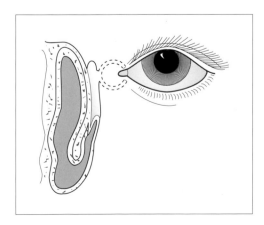

If there is persistent watering of the eye with clear fluid, the tear duct is probably blocked. No action is required until at least the age of 1 year, when the infant can be referred to an ophthalmic surgeon. Rarely, the tear duct is probed, but most ophthalmic surgeons prefer to take no action because the condition resolves spontaneously in virtually all infants and probing may induce fibrosis of the tear duct. If there is repeated or persistent purulent discharge, the possibility of chlamydia infection should be considered and arrangements made with the laboratory for specimens to be taken.

Weighing and measuring

Baby	Napkin	Vest
0–3 months	35 g	30 g
3–9 months	55 g	45 g
9–12 months	70 g	60 g

Being undressed and weighed is often the most worrying part of the visit to the child. Weighing the child in vest and napkin reduces upset and time taken. Weights of the vest and napkin should be subtracted from the total weight. Suitable scales that are checked regularly are an essential piece of equipment.

In very young infants it is easier to measure head circumference than length. The measurement should be made, using a paper tape measure, around the occipitofrontal circumference (the largest circumference). Measurements can then be plotted on a growth chart together with weights.

The length of infants aged under 2 years is measured on a special measuring board, and accurate results can be obtained only when there are two dedicated measurers present. One has to hold the infant's head against the top board while the other brings the footboard up to the child's feet while stretching him or her out. When the child is old enough to stand a special stadiometer can be used to measure height, but careful attention to detail is necessary for reproducible results.

What the newborn baby can do

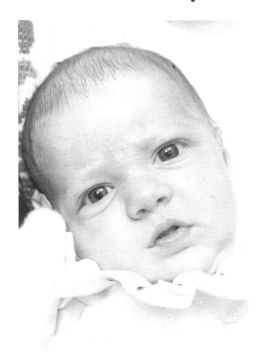

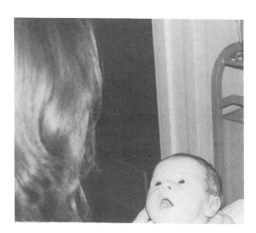

Many mothers, especially those having their first baby, believe that newborn babies are blind until they are 6 weeks old. It is not surprising that these mothers treat their babies like inanimate dolls and feel ashamed when an unexpected visitor catches them talking to the baby. The normal newborn infant can see, hear, and appreciate pain immediately after birth, even if the mother has received heavy sedation. During the hour after birth the infant is often wide awake, looking round for a feed before going to sleep or a few hours.

The distance between the eyes of the mother and the infant when the mother is breast feeding is the distance at which infants can best focus on an object. This eye to eye contact provides the first means of communication between mother and infant and is probably the reason why mothers find that covering the infants' eyes during phototherapy disturbs them. Mothers of blind infants have difficulty in feeling close to their infants. Newborn infants will become alert, frown, and gradually try to focus on a red object dangled about 12 inches before him. They stare intently at the object and will follow it with short jerking movements of the eyes if its moved slowly from side to side. Infants are also sensitive to the intensity of light and will shut their eyes tightly and keep them shut if bright light is turned on. They can discriminate shapes and patterns and the arrangements of lines from birth. They prefer patterns to dull or bright solid colours, and look longer at stripes and angles than at circular patterns.

Newborn infants can hear. They respond to sound by blinking, jerking their limbs, or drawing in breath. They may stop feeding. Mothers often speak to their infants in a high pitched voice and an infant responds more consistently to his mother's than his father's voice. An infant of 3 days of age shows preference for sweet and dislike of bitter flavoured fluid. At about the same age he can differentiate smells and distinguish between his own mother's and other mothers' breast pads.

Analysis of sound films shows that both listener and speaker are moving in time to the words of the speaker, creating a type of dance. For example, as the speaker pauses for breath or accentuates a syllable, the infant may raise an eyebrow or lower a foot. The mother notices these changes and this may encourage her to continue speaking. At a few weeks or even a few days after birth the infant may mimic gestures such as tongue protrusion, lip protrusion, or opening the mouth.

If the doctor talks to babies while examining them, mothers will not feel foolish when they do it themselves.

ACKNOWLEDGMENTS

I thank Blackwell Scientific Publications for allowing me to adapt liberally material that has appeared in *Practical Management of the Newborn, Accident and Emergency Paediatrics,* and *Paediatric Therapeutics* and use the two photographs of resuscitating a newborn.

I also thank Richard Bowlby, Joanna Fairclough, Brian Pashley, Jeanette McKenzie, Derek De Witt, and Ann Shields of the department of medical illustration at Northwick Park Hospital for taking most of the photographs. The remaining photographs were supplied as follows:

Early prenatal diagnosis: ultrasound scan, Dr H B Meire

Resuscitation of the newborn: Resuscitaire equipment, Vickers Medical.

Breathing difficulties in the newborn: micrograph of respiratory distress syndrome, Dr G Slavin; catheter electrode, Searle Medical; cerebral ultrasound, Dr R Thomas; apnoea monitor, Graesby.

Birth trauma: sternomastoid tumour from *Atlas of the Newborn* by permission of Professor Neil O'Doherty and MTP Press.

Some congenital abnormalities: cleft lip, Mr R Saunders.

Routine examination of the newborn: cardiac ultrasound, Miss Varrela Gooch.

Dislocated and dislocatable hips in the newborn: the photographs were taken by Mr E Stride.

Bacterial infection in the newborn: urine bag and suprapubic bladder puncture from *Microbial Disease* by D A J Tyrrell, Ian Phillips, C S Goodwin, and Robert Blowers by permission of the authors and Edward Arnold, publishers.

Surveillance at 8 months: distraction test from *ABC of Otolaryngology* (H Ludman), BMJ Publishing Group.

For all photographs apart from those mentioned specifically above Dr H B Valman retains the copyright.

I thank Mr R Lamont for providing extensive new material for the section on early prenatal diagnoses. I am indebted to the Child Growth Foundation for allowing the use of data to construct the growth chart on p 36, and Dr Judith Wilson for the Harrow version of the personal health record which is used for recording health surveillance data.

INDEX

Index

Index

ABCs from the BMJ

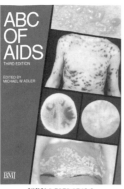
ISBN 0 7279 0761 1

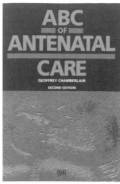
ISBN 0 7279 0884 7

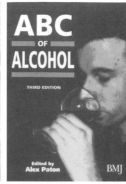
ISBN 0 7279 0794 8

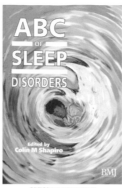
ISBN 0 7279 0812 X

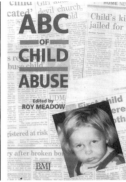
ISBN 0 7279 0764 6

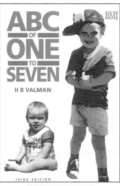
ISBN 0 7279 0768 9

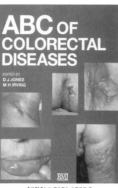
ISBN 0 7279 0755 7

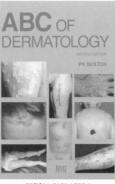
ISBN 0 7279 0777 8

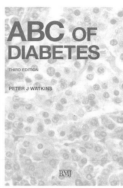
ISBN 0 7279 0763 8

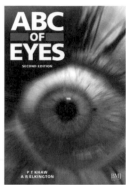
ISBN 0 7279 0766 2

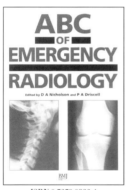
ISBN 0 7279 0832 4

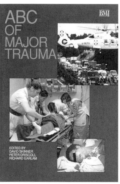
ISBN 0 7279 0291 1

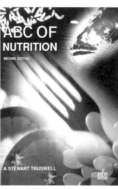
ISBN 0 7279 0315 2

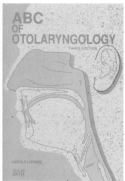
ISBN 0 7279 0765 4

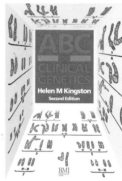
ISBN 0 7279 0846 4

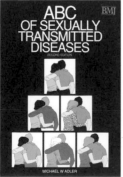
ISBN 0 7279 0261 X

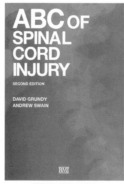
ISBN 0 7279 0760 3

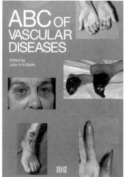
ISBN 0 7279 0754 9

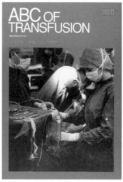
ISBN 0 7279 0259 8

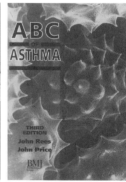
ISBN 0 7279 0882 0

For further details contact your local bookseller or write to:

BMJ Publishing Group
BMA House
Tavistock Square
London WC1H 9JR (U.K.)

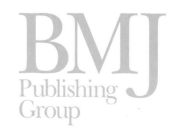